Towards the Eradication of *Helicobacter pylori* Infection - Rapid Diagnosis and Precision Treatment

Edited by Liang Wang, Alfred Chin Yen Tay and Barry J. Marshall

Published in London, United Kingdom

Towards the Eradication of *Helicobacter pylori* Infection - Rapid Diagnosis and Precision Treatment
http://dx.doi.org/10.5772/intechopen.111873
Edited by Liang Wang, Alfred Chin Yen Tay and Barry J. Marshall

Contributors
Andrea Muiño, Annabel E. Barber, Chiara Della Bella, Guo-Xin Zhang, Harry Hua-Xiang Xia, He Haolong, Isabel Adler, Jing Zhang, Joy Qing-Jiao Liao, Ka Shing Cheung, Liu Mi, Liu Weiai, Lok Ka Lam, Mario M. D'Elios, Meiling Zhou, Pablo Rodríguez, She Chang, Shigang Ding, Taylor Fontenot, Valeria Denninghoff, Weiguang Qiao, Weiwei Fu, Xiao-Ying Zhou, Xu Xuan, Yu Chen, Zhou Jingying

First published in London, United Kingdom, 2024 by IntechOpen
IntechOpen is the global imprint of INTECHOPEN LIMITED, registered in England and Wales, registration number: 11086078, 167-169 Great Portland Street, London, W1W 5PF, United Kingdom

British Library Cataloguing-in-Publication Data
A catalogue record for this book is available from the British Library

Additional hard and PDF copies can be obtained from orders@intechopen.com

Towards the Eradication of *Helicobacter pylori* Infection - Rapid Diagnosis and Precision Treatment
Edited by Liang Wang, Alfred Chin Yen Tay and Barry J. Marshall
p. cm.
Print ISBN 978-0-85466-446-7
Online ISBN 978-0-85466-445-0
eBook (PDF) ISBN 978-0-85466-447-4

Meet the editors

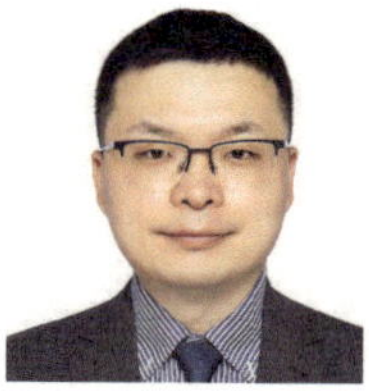

Liang Wang is a professor and a group leader (principal investigator) at Guangdong Provincial People's Hospital (Guangdong Academy of Medical Sciences), Southern Medical University, China. He also works as a research fellow at the University of Queensland and the University of Western Australia. He is an adjunct professor at the School of Medical and Health Sciences, Edith Cowan University, Australia. His current research interests are computational and experimental bacteriology, focusing on bacterial evolution, metabolism, and rapid diagnosis. Prof. Wang serves as an associate editor for *Frontiers in Microbiology* and is an editorial board member of *BMC Bioinformatics, PeerJ, Heliyon*, and others. To date, Prof. Wang has published more than 100 peer-reviewed papers in international journals.

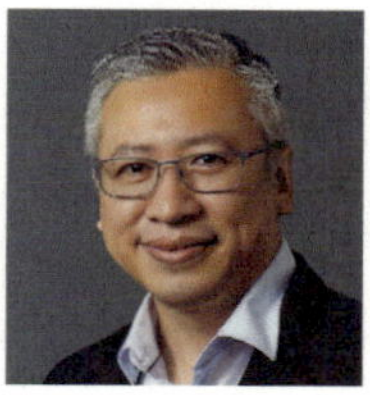

Alfred Chin Yen Tay is a leading researcher in *H. pylori* epidemiology, studying *Helicobacter* diversity in humans and animals through genomic analysis. His work at the Helicobacter Research Laboratory in the UWA Marshall Centre for Infectious Diseases Research and Training focuses on developing new diagnostic tools for *Helicobacter* infection. Dr. Tay's studies on *H. pylori* antibiotic resistance have led to improved diagnostics and personalized treatments, achieving a 90% cure rate for resistant cases. He also founded the Helicobacter Fellowship Training Program, supported by the Australia Department of Foreign Affairs and Trading (DFAT), to enhance *H. pylori* research in developing countries. Dr. Tay is passionate about reducing the global gastric cancer rate by supporting local *H. pylori* research in these nations.

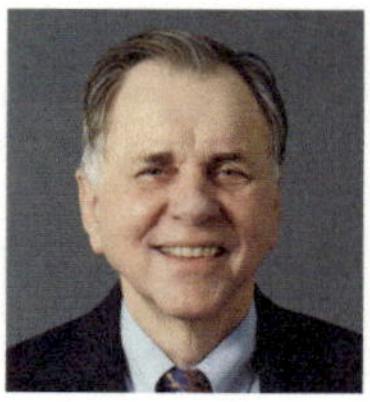

Barry J. Marshall has managed a *Helicobacter pylori* research group almost since he discovered *Helicobacter pylori* with Robin Warren in 1982. Prof. Marshall received many honors for his work on *Helicobacter pylori*, most notably the Nobel Prize for Medicine or Physiology in 2005. In the past few years, Prof. Marshall's laboratory has developed enhanced methods for noninvasive studies on the molecular epidemiology of *H. pylori*, notably a rapid breath test and retrieval of the organism (and culture) from a swallowed string. Prof. Marshall has recently succeeded in drawing investor funding from international and national sources for the creation of Ondek, a small biotech company focused on developing new biologic delivery systems for vaccines and therapeutics, utilizing genetically modified *Helicobacter pylori*.

Contents

Watch editors' insights by scanning this QR code.

Preface

The persistent presence of *Helicobacter pylori* (*H. pylori*) infection poses a significant challenge to global public health. Despite decades of research and medical advancements, eradication of the bacterium remains elusive in many cases. The urgency to address this issue has led to a multidisciplinary approach, integrating rapid diagnosis and precision treatment strategies. This book, *Towards the Eradication of* Helicobacter pylori *Infection – Rapid Diagnosis and Precision Treatment*, serves as a comprehensive guide to navigating through the complexities of diagnosing and treating *H. pylori* infection.

The first part of this book delves into the various diagnostic modalities available for identifying *H. pylori* infection. In particular, Chapter 1 provides insights into rapid, noninvasive techniques for detecting antibiotic resistance, a crucial aspect in tailoring effective treatment regimens. Chapter 2 elucidates the roles of key cytokines, interleukin 17 and interferon-gamma, in inflammation and diagnosis of *H. pylori* and associated gastric malignancies. Chapter 3 offers a thorough review of invasive methods employed in diagnosing *H. pylori* infection, highlighting current practices and their clinical implications. Finally, Chapter 4 explores the utility of linked color imaging in endoscopic diagnosis, offering advancements in visualizing *H. pylori*-associated lesions.

Furthermore, the second part of this book shifts the focus toward treating *H. pylori* infection, addressing the challenges posed by antibiotic resistance and the role of stewardship in optimizing treatment outcomes. Chapter 5 navigates through antibiotic resistance patterns, emphasizing the importance of susceptibility testing and stewardship programs in guiding therapeutic decisions. Chapter 6 expands the horizon by examining the relationship between *H. pylori* infection and oral pathology, shedding light on potential oral manifestations and implications for treatment. Chapter 7 delves into the dynamic changes of host immune response during *H. pylori*-induced gastric carcinogenesis, providing insights into novel immunotherapeutic approaches. Finally, Chapter 8 explores complementary replacement therapy as a potential adjunctive treatment for chronic gastritis, offering a holistic approach to managing *H. pylori*-related gastric inflammation.

This book amalgamates cutting-edge research, clinical insights, and practical applications, aiming to equip healthcare professionals, researchers, and students with the knowledge and tools necessary to combat *H. pylori* infection effectively. As we embark on this journey toward eradication, it is imperative to harness collective expertise across various disciplines to achieve our ultimate goal of eliminating the burden of *H. pylori*-associated diseases. May this comprehensive compendium stand as a testament to the relentless pursuit of understanding and combating *H. pylori* infection, offering a multifaceted exploration of diagnostic modalities, therapeutic interventions, and emerging strategies aimed at its eradication. As we navigate the intricate landscape of *H. pylori*-associated diseases, this scholarly tome endeavors to illuminate the path toward effective management and mitigation of its deleterious effects on human health. Through the meticulous elucidation of molecular mechanisms, epidemiological trends, and clinical outcomes, this collective endeavor seeks to arm clinicians, researchers, and public health practitioners with the requisite knowledge and tools to confront this formidable pathogen. By fostering interdisciplinary collaboration and fostering the dissemination of cutting-edge research findings, this volume endeavors to catalyze transformative advancements in the field, ultimately envisioning a future liberated from the burdens of *H. pylori* infection.

Finally, we are honored to extend my deepest gratitude to all the esteemed authors who contributed their invaluable insights and expertise to this book. Their dedication and scholarly contributions have truly enriched the content and advanced the discourse within its pages. We would also like to express our heartfelt appreciation to Mr. Josip Knapić, whose diligent efforts as the publishing process manager ensured the smooth execution of this project. His guidance and support were instrumental in bringing this endeavor to fruition. Additionally, we extend our sincere thanks to IntechOpen, the world's leading publisher of Open Access books, for their commitment to advancing scientific knowledge and fostering collaboration within the academic community.

Liang Wang
Department of Laboratory Medicine,
Guangdong Provincial People's Hospital,
Guangdong Academy of Medical Sciences,
Southern Medical University,
Guangzhou, China

Alfred Chin Yen Tay
Helicobacter pylori Research Laboratory,
Marshall Centre for Infectious Disease Research and Training,
School of Biomedical Sciences,
Faculty of Health and Medical Sciences,
The University of Western Australia,
Perth, Australia

Barry J. Marshall
Helicobacter pylori Research Laboratory,
Marshall Centre for Infectious Disease Research and Training,
School of Biomedical Sciences,
Faculty of Health and Medical Sciences,
The University of Western Australia,
Perth, Australia

Marshall Laboratory of Biomedical Engineering,
School of Biomedical Engineering,
Shenzhen University, Shenzhen,
Guangdong, China

Section 1

Diagnosis of *Helicobacter pylori* Infection

Chapter 1

Rapid Non-Invasive Techniques for Detecting Antibiotic Resistance in *Helicobacter pylori*: An Update and Clinical Applications

Xiao-Ying Zhou, Guo-Xin Zhang, Joy Qing-Jiao Liao and Harry Hua-Xiang Xia

Abstract

The global prevalence of *Helicobacter pylori* infection remains high, posing a significant health challenge worldwide. The efficacy of anti-*H. pylori* antibiotic-based regimens is compromised by the increasing antibiotic resistance in *H. pylori*. Thus, it is important to detect antibiotic resistance in *H. pylori* to ensure appropriate and effective treatment strategies. Currently, conventional culture-based methods are used for detecting antibiotic resistance (so-called phenotypic resistance) in *H. pylori*, but these methods are tedious and time-consuming (at least 72 h) and rely on the successful culture of *H. pylori*. Over the past decade, emerging genotypic or molecular techniques based on polymerase chain reaction or gene sequencing of DNA extracted from cultured *H. pylori* cells or *H. pylori*-containing specimens, such as gastric biopsy, stool, or saliva, have been developed to detect antibiotic resistance (so-called genotypic resistance) in *H. pylori*. These methods are rapid (usually within 4 h), non- or minimally invasive, cost-effective, and highly reproducible. Moreover, they can detect heteroresistant strains, enabling tailored therapy. The development and implementation of molecular techniques have significantly improved the accuracy and speed of identifying antibiotic resistance in *H. pylori*, allowing for more effective and personalized treatment strategies.

Keywords: *Helicobacter pylori*, antibiotic resistance, antibiotic susceptibility testing, rapid non-invasive technique, tailored therapy

1. Introduction

Helicobacter pylori is a gram-negative bacterium that colonizes the human stomach, affecting approximately half of the global population [1]. *H. pylori* infection is not only a major cause of various gastrointestinal diseases, including gastritis, peptic ulcers, mucosa-associated lymphoid tissue lymphoma, and gastric cancer but also associated with various extra-gastrointestinal diseases, such as diabetes mellitus,

IntechOpen

idiopathic thrombocytopenic purpura, *etc*. [2]. It has been established that eradication of *H. pylori* infection is crucial for the treatment and prevention of these diseases. Currently recommended *H. pylori* eradication regimens include triple therapies containing a proton pump inhibitor such as omeprazole/esomeprazole, lansoprazole or pantoprazole, or vonoprazan and two of the following antibiotics including metronidazole, amoxicillin, clarithromycin, tetracycline, levofloxacin, or quadruple therapies containing a proton pump inhibitor, a bismuth salt, and two of the above-mentioned antibiotics [3]. Clinically, these regimens usually initially achieved eradication rates of over 85% [4]. However, the emergence and spread of antibiotic resistance among *H. pylori* strains significantly affects the clinical efficacy of these triple or quadruple regimens, thus becoming major challenges in achieving successful eradication. Although vonoprazan appears to regain the efficacy of triple therapies, vonoprazan-containing triple therapies are reported to contribute to antibiotic resistance if treatment fails [5, 6]. Therefore, identifying antibiotic resistance in *H. pylori* is important for specifically selecting antibiotics for the eradication of *H. pylori* infection.

Currently, conventional culture-based microbiological methods are commonly used to determine the susceptibility of *H. pylori* strains to various recommended antibiotics [7–11]. However, these methods are tedious, time-consuming, costly, and, more importantly, invasive. In addition, culture of *H. pylori* from gastric biopsies is not always successful due to technical difficulty, and thus susceptibility testing results may not be available for some patients with *H. pylori* infection. Therefore, a rapid, non-invasive, and accurate technique for the determination of susceptibility of *H. pylori* to antibiotics is required for specific targeting treatment of the infection. At present, several rapid, mostly non-invasive, techniques for determining the susceptibility of *H. pylori* to antibiotics have been explored [12–20]. This chapter aims to emphasize the importance of detecting antibiotic resistance in *H. pylori*, describe currently used conventional methods and particularly emerging rapid non-invasive techniques for detecting antibiotic resistance in *H. pylori* and their clinical implications, and propose future research directions.

2. Importance of detecting antibiotic resistance in *H. pylori*

Antibiotic resistance refers to the ability of bacteria to survive and multiply in the presence of antibiotics which would normally inhibit or kill them. The development of antibiotic resistance in *H. pylori* is primarily attributed to the overuse and misuse of antibiotics in clinical practice.

The clinical efficacy of currently recommended eradication treatment regimens heavily relies on the susceptibility of *H. pylori* strains to antibiotics. Early studies have demonstrated that primary or secondary (acquired) resistance leads to treatment failure [21, 22] and the persistence or recrudescence of *H. pylori* infection is associated with chronic or recurrent diseases associated with *H. pylori* infection [23]. The impact of antibiotic resistance on the success rate of eradication therapies has been confirmed by recent studies. For instance, Wong *et al*. showed that metronidazole resistance was associated with a decreased response to metronidazole-containing regimens; the eradication rate was 87.2 and 67.6% ($P = 0.001$) for patients with metronidazole sensitive and resistant isolates, respectively [24]. Similarly, Arenas *et al.* found that clarithromycin resistance significantly reduced the eradication rate of *H. pylori* when using clarithromycin-based regimens (OR: 0.13; 95% confidence interval, 0.04–0.49) [25].

The effects of antibiotic resistance on the clinical efficacy of *H. pylori* eradication regimens are not limited to these two antibiotics. Resistance to other commonly used antibiotics, such as amoxicillin, levofloxacin, and tetracycline, has also been reported to compromise the success of eradication therapies [26–28]. Thus, *H. pylori* eradication should be guided by antibiotic susceptibility testing (AST), preferably by genotypic methods. Indeed, a recent meta-analysis enrolled 12 qualified randomized controlled trials containing 3940 patients clearly demonstrated that the pooled eradication rates of tailored therapy based on the detection of genotypic resistance were consistently higher than those in the empirical treatment group [29].

Therefore, to ensure the efficacy of *H. pylori* eradication therapies, it is essential to detect antibiotic resistance in *H. pylori* before initiating treatment. By identifying the antibiotic susceptibility profile of *H. pylori*, clinicians can tailor the treatment regimens to the individual patients.

3. Conventional phenotypic culture-based methods for detecting antibiotic resistance in *H. pylori* and their limitations

The conventional microbiological methods are mainly based on the culture of the gastric biopsies taken during upper endoscopy, subculture of *H. pylori* colonies, and observation of the ability of the *H. pylori* isolates to grow on agar plates containing various concentrations of antibiotics, and measurements of the minimal inhibitory concentrations (MIC) or the minimal diameter of the inhibitory zone (MID) [7, 8]; the cut-off MICs and MIDs of commonly used antibiotics are listed in **Table 1**. Thus, these methods directly determine the phenotypic pattern of antibiotic susceptibility of *H. pylori* and are thus considered to be accurate in detecting antibiotic resistance (or specifically phenotypic antibiotic resistance) in *H. pylori*.

Currently, four phenotypic methods including the agar dilution method, broth microdilution method, disk diffusion test, and the Epsilometer test (or the E-test) are commonly used in clinical practice [7–9].

Antibiotic	The cut-off MIC (μg/mL) differentiating susceptibility and resistance	The cut-off MID (cm) differentiating susceptibility and resistance
Metronidazole	>8.0 [7, 30–34]	<20 (5 μg/disk) [7]
Clarithromycin	>0.5 [31–35] or 1.0 [19] or 2.0 [36]	<30 (15 μg/disk) [36]
Tetracycline	>1.0 [31–35]	
Amoxicillin	>0.125 [31, 33, 34], 0.25 [32] or 0.5 [35]	
Levofloxacin	>0.5 [35] or 1.0 [31–34]	
Rifampicin	>1.0 [31, 32, 34]	
Rifabutin	>1.0 [33]	
Furazolidone	>2.0 [32]	<21 (100 μg/disk) [31, 37]

The cut-off criteria are mainly derived from EUCAST [34].
MIC, the minimal inhibitory concentration as detected by the agar dilution method, or the Epsilometer test (or the E-test); MID, the minimal diameter of the inhibitory zone as detected by the disk diffusion test.

Table 1.
The cut-off minimal inhibitory concentrations and the minimal diameter of the inhibitory zones differentiating susceptibility and resistance in Helicobacter pylori *to various commonly used antibiotics.*

- *Agar dilution method*

  The agar dilution method is considered the gold standard for detecting bacterial susceptibility to antibiotics and is recommended by the Clinical and Laboratory Standard Institute (CLSI). Briefly, bacterial suspension (2.0 McFarland) of each of multiple *H. pylori* strains or isolates is spot-inoculated on Mueller-Hinton or chocolate agar in a 150 mm plate; the agar medium is supplemented with 5 to 10% sheep or horse blood and contains one of 2-fold dilution concentrations of an antibiotic. The agar plates are incubated at 35–37°C in a microaerophilic environment and read for bacterial growth after 72 h of incubation. The lowest antibiotic concentration at which there is no growth is defined as the MIC of the antibiotic for the tested *H. pylori* strain or isolate [7, 8].

- *Broth microdilution method*

  Similar to the agar dilution method, this method involves the preparation of serial dilutions of antibiotics in a liquid growth medium. *H. pylori* suspension is added to each well containing one of the antibiotic dilutions, and the MIC is determined as the lowest concentration of the antibiotic that inhibits bacterial growth. This method is now increasingly used in epidemiological studies and clinical practice [9].

- *Disk diffusion method*

  The disk diffusion method, or Kirby-Bauer test, is commonly used in epidemiological studies. Briefly, a standardized inoculum is swabbed onto the surface of Mueller-Hinton or chocolate agar in a 150 mm plate. Then, filter paper disks impregnated with standardized concentrations of a few different antibiotics are placed on the surface of predefined areas. The plates are incubated as described for the agar dilution method, and the size of the zone of inhibition around each of the disks is measured after 72 h [7, 10]. However, this method has a labor-intensive nature stemming from manual measurements and data documentation, and mainly relies on investigator skill, leading to potential variations in results [38, 39].

- *E-test*

  This method is also known as the Epsilometer test. It employs a bacterial solution calibrated to the McFarland standard of 3.0 on Muller-Hinton agar supplemented with 5–10% sheep blood. Under microaerophilic circumstances, an E-test strip impregnated with escalating quantities of antibiotics is placed on inoculation plates and incubated for 72 hours at a temperature of 37°C. The MIC is provided by an elliptical zone of inhibition. When compared to the agar dilution or broth dilution procedures, the E-test is straightforward to execute, and the results have been found to correlate closely with results obtained by the gold standard (agar dilution), except for metronidazole, for which recent studies have revealed inconsistency in the results [11]. The E-test possesses all the disadvantages that the disk diffusion method does [7, 10, 11].

The above-described culture-based conventional phenotypic AST methods provide valuable and accurate information on the susceptibility of *H. pylori* to antibiotics. However, they have several limitations. First, the commonly used specimens for isolation and culture of *H. pylori* are gastric biopsies taken during the upper endoscopy. Thus, upper endoscopic examination is a prerequisite for most cases. Noticeably, upper endoscopy is an invasive procedure that does not apply to the general population. Second, isolation and subculture of *H. pylori* are difficult due to the finicky nature of the bacterium and the high possibility of contamination with commensals, and thus, AST of *H. pylori* can be carried out only in well-equipped laboratories with well-trained technicians. In addition, sufficient live *H. pylori* bacterial cells in the specimen are required for successful isolation of the bacterium. Inadequate or delayed specimen handling and processing and recent exposure to antibiotics or proton pump inhibitors (PPIs) would reduce the number of live *H. pylori* and thus decrease the success rates [40, 41]. Indeed, the success rates for isolation of *H. pylori* from gastric biopsies range from 67.9 to 96.0% in clinical practice [41, 42]. Finally, all culture-based conventional phenotypic methods are tedious and time-consuming as they all require a long (at least 72 h) cultural procedure and rely on the successful isolation and subculture of the *H. pylori* isolate.

4. Genotypic or molecular-based methods for detecting antibiotic resistance in *H. pylori* and their clinical applications

Given the limitations of conventional phenotypic methods, there is a pressing need for rapid non-invasive techniques for detecting antibiotic resistance in *H. pylori*. It has been revealed that antibiotic resistance in *H. pylori* is primarily attributed to point mutations in specific genes; the point mutations rendering the resistance in *H. pylori* to antibiotics commonly used in clinical practice are summarized in **Table 2**. Therefore, genotypic or molecular methods that are based on polymerase chain reaction (PCR) or gene sequencing of DNA extracted from purely cultured *H. pylori* cells or *H. pylori*-containing specimens, such as gastric biopsy, stool, or saliva, have emerged to detect antibiotic resistance (or specifically genotypic resistance) in *H. pylori*. These methods are non- or minimally invasive, more rapid (usually within 4 h), cost-effective, highly reproducible, and less affected by the modulation of bacterial burden caused by the recent use of antibiotics and PPIs [12–20, 56–75]. Moreover, they can

Antibiotic	Drug class	Resistance mechanism	Mutation position
Metronidazole [43, 44]	Nitroimidazole	Insertions/deletions, frameshift mutations or missense and premature truncations in *rdxA* gene	
Clarithromycin [43, 45, 46]	Macrolide	The V domain of *23S rRNA*	A2142G, A2143G, A2142C
Tetracycline [47–49]	Tetracycline	Triple base pair substitutions of 16S rRNA	Positions 926–928
Amoxicillin [50, 51]	β-lactam	Mutations in *pbp1A* gene	
Levofloxacin [52, 53]	Fluoroquinolone	The QRDR within *gyrA* gene	Codons 87 and 91
Rifampicin [54, 55]	Rifamycin	Point mutations in the RRDR of *rpoB* gene	Codons 525 to 545, 547, and 586

Table 2.
The genetic mechanisms rendering the resistance in Helicobacter pylori *to various antibiotics commonly used in clinical practice.*

detect heteroresistant strains, which enables tailored therapy [41, 73, 74, 76, 77]. Therefore, genotypic methods can be used as an alternative to culture-based methods for detecting the resistance in *H. pylori* to various antibiotics.

Several molecular-based methods, mainly based on PCR and sequencing, including allele-specific PCR (AS-PCR), real-time quantitative PCR (RT-qPCR), multiplex PCR, nested PCR, digital PCR (dPCR), and next-generation sequencing (NGS) have been developed to detect genotypic resistance in *H. pylori* [12–20, 56–75]. The methods detect mutations either by polymorphic or mutant allele-directed specific analysis using specific primers or melting curve analysis [78]. In addition, the fluorescence *in situ* hybridization (FISH) technique has also been applied to detect antibiotic heteroresistant strains of *H. pylori* [73, 74].

4.1 PCR-based methods

4.1.1 Allele-specific PCR (AS-PCR)

This method involves designing specific primers that target known resistance-associated mutations in genes responsible for antibiotic resistance. By amplifying the target region, the presence or absence of specific mutations can be determined. AS-PCR is applied by performing PCR using primers specific to the target mutation(s) and analyzing the resulting PCR products to identify the presence of resistance-associated mutations [12].

4.2 Real-time quantitative PCR (RT-qPCR)

This technique allows for the quantification of DNA in real-time during the amplification process. It can be used to detect the presence of specific antibiotic resistance genes or mutations in *H. pylori*. RT-qPCR is applied by designing primers and a fluorescent probe specific to the target gene or mutation. The amplification is monitored in real-time using a fluorescent signal, and the presence or absence of the target sequence is determined based on the amplification curve [13, 17–19]. Currently, a few commercial RT-qPCR kits that detect clarithromycin resistance in *H. pylori*, namely, ClariRes RT-PCR, Lightmix RT-PCR, and TaqMan RT-PCR, are available [56–61]. These methods are reported to produce high concordance or accuracy rates (>90%), compared with the E-test [44].

4.3 Multiplex PCR

This method enables the simultaneous amplification of multiple target genes or regions in a single reaction. It can be used to detect multiple antibiotic-resistance genes or mutations in *H. pylori*. Multiplex PCR is applied by designing primers specific to each target gene or mutation and optimizing the reaction conditions to ensure efficient amplification of all targets in a single reaction [14–16].

4.4 Nested PCR

This method involves two rounds of PCR amplification, with the second round using primers that are specific to the product of the first round. It can be used to increase the sensitivity and specificity of detecting antibiotic-resistance genes or mutations in *H. pylori*. Nested PCR is applied by performing an initial PCR using outer primers that amplify the target region, followed by a second PCR using inner primers that specifically amplify the product from the first round. The resulting PCR products are then analyzed to detect the presence of resistance-associated genes or mutations [20].

4.5 Digital PCR

Digital PCR partitions the PCR reaction into thousands of individual reactions, allowing for the absolute quantification of target DNA molecules. This technique has been explored to detect and quantify low-abundance antibiotic resistance mutations in *H. pylori* [62]. Specifically, a droplet digital PCR assay was established to detect *H. pylori* clarithromycin resistance-related 23S rRNA alleles in gastric and stool samples. Of the gastric samples of 46 patients, 22 (48%) had only wild-type (clarithromycin susceptible) alleles, and 24 (52%) had clarithromycin resistance alleles. Of the 24 with clarithromycin resistance alleles, 11 had clarithromycin resistance alleles only, and 13 had a mixed population of clarithromycin resistance and wild-type alleles, suggesting heteroresistance. Of the stool samples of 45 patients, 17 (38%) had only wild-type (clarithromycin susceptible) alleles, and 28 (62%) had clarithromycin resistance alleles. Of the 28 with clarithromycin resistance alleles, 11 had only clarithromycin resistance alleles, and 17 had a mixed population of clarithromycin resistance and wild-type alleles. The dPCR results were highly concordant with that of culture E-test results [62].

4.5.1 Sequencing-based methods

Next-generation sequencing (NGS) techniques have evolved into potent, quick (turnaround time of 24–72 h), and cost-effective methods for predicting antibiotic resistance in *H. pylori* [63]. They can evaluate several genes at the same time. NGS techniques are highly sensitive for detecting the presence of mutations and resistance genes, compared with PCR-based techniques which only detect specific target genes, and thus can lead to false negatives. The commonly used NGS technique is whole-genome sequencing (WGS), which allows the determination of the entire DNA sequence of an organism, and thus the presence or absence of certain genes and single-nucleotide polymorphisms (SNPs) that are associated with or responsible for antibiotic resistance [64–67]. This method can be used to directly guide the treatment for individual patients and to indirectly establish treatment guidelines according to the local pattern of antibiotic resistance [64]. At present, the WGS technique has already been applied directly to *H. pylori* resistance to antibiotics not only with cultured *H. pylori* bacterial cells but also with clinical specimens, providing an attractive option [68, 69].

Another NGS technique that has been explored to detect antibiotic resistance in *H. pylori* is ChIP-sequencing, a gene chip technique. Based on the principle of complementary pairing of bases, this technique is reported to have high sensitivity, specificity, and high-throughput capacity for detecting antibiotic resistance of *H. pylori* directly from gastric biopsies. Yin *et al.* used ChIP-sequencing to rapidly diagnose *H. pylori* infection and detect antibiotic-resistant *H. pylori* in children. They found that the sensitivity, specificity, and accuracy of the gene chip technology for diagnosing *H. pylori* infection were 96.1, 85.0, and 93.6%, respectively. Moreover, they identified several main *H. pylori* resistance gene loci using the gene chip; the main mutation loci were 2143A/G for clarithromycin, GyrA 91 and GyrA 87 for levofloxacin, and PBP1 556ser for amoxicillin. Concordance rates between the gene chip technique and DNA sequencing were greater than 95% for VacA-S/M, 16S rRNA, 23S rRNA, and GyrA, and greater than 82% for PBP1 [70].

Other NGS techniques, including whole exome sequencing, methyl sequencing, targeted resequencing, *de novo* sequencing, and RNA sequencing [71, 72], may be also applied in the detection of antibiotic resistance in *H. pylori* although their values have not yet been explored.

4.5.2 FISH

This technique has also been applied to detect antibiotic heteroresistant strains of *H. pylori* [73, 74]. Kocsmár *et al*. used an rRNA-targeted clarithromycin resistance FISH test for the antral and corpus biopsy specimens of 305 *H. pylori*-infected patients. They detected clarithromycin-resistant *H. pylori* in 73 (23.9%) cases, which consisted of 35 (11.5%) homoresistant and 38 (12.5%) heteroresistant cases [73]. They further used the same technique to investigate the proportion of resistant bacteria in the bacterial population (R-fraction) and its predictive role for the use of clarithromycin-based therapies in patients with clarithromycin-heteroresistant *H. pylori* infection. They observed that the R-fraction was significantly increased in patients with multiple previous eradication attempts, including at least one clarithromycin-containing therapy than in those with only one previous eradication attempt. In addition, multivariable regression analysis showed that the therapeutic outcome using clarithromycin-based regimens depended on the bacterial density, not a high R-fraction [74], suggesting the potential re-use of clarithromycin-containing regimens in patients with clarithromycin-heteroresistant *H. pylori* infection. However, a high bacterial density is prone to the acquisition of antibiotic resistance during the treatment, which is likely to be the actual cause of the treatment failure [75].

4.5.3 Clinical applications of genotypic or molecular-based methods

The use of molecular-based methods for detecting antibiotic resistance in *H. pylori* has revolutionized the management approach for patients with *H. pylori* infection. By providing rapid and accurate results, these methods enable clinicians to prescribe the most effective antibiotic regimen, thereby increasing the chances of successful eradication and reducing the spread of resistant strains. In two large randomized controlled trials of 880 patients (560 eligible treatment-naive and 320 with refractory *H pylori* infection), Chen *et al.* demonstrated that clinical efficacy as represented by the eradication rate was comparable between the molecular method-guided therapy and culture-based method-guided therapy when used as the first-line therapy and rescue treatment of *H. pylori* infection, hence supporting the use of molecular method-guided therapy for *H. pylori* eradication [79]. More recently, Li *et al.* reported that genotypic antibiotic resistance-tailored bismuth-containing quadruple therapy resulted in eradication rates of 87.1 and 95.8% by intention-to-treat (ITT) analysis and per-protocol (PP) analysis, respectively [80]. Lin *et al.* reported that, in a meta-analysis of 4626 patients, the pooled eradication rates of the first-line and rescue genotypic antibiotic resistance-tailored therapies were 86.6 and 85.1% by ITT analysis and 92.0 and 87.9% by PP analysis, respectively. When tailored rescue therapy was based on the genotypic resistance to at least four antibiotics, the pooled eradication rates reached 89.4% by ITT analysis and 92.1% by PP analysis. For genotype-susceptible strains, the pooled eradication rate with targeted antibiotics was 93.1%

(95% CI:91.3–94.9%) [81]. Moreover, a recent meta-analysis demonstrated that molecular method-guided therapy is more efficacious than empirical therapy when used as triple therapy (not as quadruple therapy) [29].

Despite numerous advantages, molecular-based methods have limitations. PCR- or NGS-based techniques are incapable of determining MIC, and the contribution of each mutation to the MIC is not always obvious. Moreover, genomic prediction of resistance and phenotypic culture-based susceptibility testing do not always correspond. In addition, molecular-based methods can also underestimate resistance caused by non-genetic mechanisms. Therefore, there is a need for additional research to determine which genes or gene involvement patterns correlate most strongly with phenotypic outcomes. To overcome the diminished predictive value that could be the result of DNA fragmentation in formalin-fixed paraffin-embedded tissue samples or associated contamination in stool samples, excellent DNA extraction methods need to be developed. Consequently, studies with broader gene coverages, larger sample sizes, or multicenter designs from various geographic regions are necessary. Moreover, standardized and user-friendly computational software and tools must be developed so that data obtained from molecular-based methods, especially NGS, can be easily analyzed and implemented in routine clinical settings.

Taken together, molecular-based methods have emerged as valuable tools for detecting antibiotic resistance in *H. pylori*. They offer rapid and accurate results, enabling effective patient management. However, continuous research is needed to improve these methods and overcome their limitations.

4.5.4 Novel techniques for collecting specimens for genotypic-based methods for detecting antibiotic resistance in H. pylori

Specimens currently used for detecting genotypic resistance of *H. pylori* include gastric biopsy, stool, or saliva [57, 61, 76]. Recently, Han *et al.* evaluated a string-test kit for the collection of gastric material, on which RT-qPCR was performed for the detection of *H. pylori* infection and genotypic resistance to clarithromycin and levofloxacin. They demonstrated that there was a concordance rate of 95.9% between such a string-qPCR and ^{13}C-urea breath test, an accurate non-invasive method widely used in clinical practice for diagnosis of *H. pylori* infection. Moreover, they reported a high eradication rate of 91.8% with genotypic resistance-tailored bismuth quadruple therapy [82]. The value of the string test coupled with RT-qPCR for detecting *H. pylori* resistance to clarithromycin and levofloxacin has also been validated in urban China in a recent multicenter, cross-sectional study [83]. Therefore, the string-qPCR test is a feasible method that can facilitate the detection of genotypic antibiotic resistance in *H. pylori*, and thus further improve the clinical practice in the treatment of *H. pylori* infection. The detailed procedures of the string-qPCR test are presented as a video demonstration in a recent publication [84]. In addition, Tang *et al.* evaluated surface-enhanced Raman spectroscopy (SERS) in combination with machine learning algorithms for the detection of *H. pylori* infection in human gastric fluid samples collected with the string test. They found that this novel technique achieved a prediction accuracy of 82.2% in the detection of *H. pylori* infection [85]; however, the value of SERS coupled with machine learning algorithms in detecting genotypic antibiotic resistance in *H. pylori* needs to be further investigated.

5. Future research directions

The global prevalence of *H. pylori* infection remains high, posing a significant health burden. However, current antibiotic treatment strategies are not entirely effective due to increasing antibiotic resistance. Therefore, there is an urgent need to optimize antibiotic-based therapies or to explore novel non-antibiotic therapeutic approaches.

First, future research should focus on the optimization of antibiotic-based therapies. On the one hand, antibiotic resistance-tailored therapy should be applied where feasible. The recent Maastricht VI Consensus recommends that second-line and rescue therapies be guided by local resistance patterns as determined by susceptibility testing and monitoring eradication rates to maximize treatment success [86]. With the advent of molecular techniques, rapid, non- or minimally invasive, accurate detection of antibiotic resistance in *H. pylori* will be readily available soon. Well-designed randomized controlled trials that include a large number of cases and compare AST-guided rescue therapy with empirical rescue therapy should be carried out to achieve optimized antibiotic-based therapies. On the other hand, further research is needed to evaluate the efficacy of newly claimed promising empirical medicines, such as vonoprazan-based therapies [4, 5, 87], with susceptibility-guided therapy.

Besides antibiotic therapeutic targets, future research should also focus on understanding the molecular mechanisms of *H. pylori* pathogenesis and host immune response, which could lead to the development of targeted therapies and vaccines. For example, a recent animal study by Liu *et al*. explored a nanoparticle-based sonodynamic therapy, that effectively neutralizes vacuolating cytotoxin A, a key virulence factor secreted by *H. pylori*, and generates reactive oxygen species. It was observed that this non-antibiotic approach reduced *H. pylori* infection in mice without disrupting gut microbiota, and thus could be an alternative to antibiotic-based therapies for *H. pylori* infection [88]. However, its clinical relevance needs to be verified.

Author details

Xiao-Ying Zhou[1,2], Guo-Xin Zhang[1,2], Joy Qing-Jiao Liao[3] and
Harry Hua-Xiang Xia[3,4]*

1 Department of Gastroenterology, First Affiliated Hospital of Nanjing Medical University, Nanjing, China

2 First Clinical Medical College of Nanjing Medical University, Nanjing, China

3 Medjaden Inc. Wuhan, China

4 Department of Gastroenterology, The First Affiliated Hospital of Guangdong Pharmaceutical University, Guangzhou, China

*Address all correspondence to: xiaharry@hotmail.com

References

[1] Hooi JKY, Lai WY, Ng WK, Suen MMY, Underwood FE, Tanyingoh D, et al. Global prevalence of *Helicobacter pylori* infection: Systematic review and meta-analysis. Gastroenterology. 2017;**153**(2):420-429

[2] Pellicano R, Ianiro G, Fagoonee S, Settanni CR, Gasbarrini A. Review: Extragastric diseases and *Helicobacter pylori*. Helicobacter. 2020;**25**(Suppl. 1): e12741

[3] Bujanda L, Nyssen OP, Ramos J, Bordin DS, Tepes B, Perez-Aisa A, et al. Effectiveness of *Helicobacter pylori* treatments according to antibiotic resistance. The American Journal of Gastroenterology. 2024:**119**(4):646-654

[4] Zhou BG, Jiang X, Ding YB, She Q, Li YY. Vonoprazan-amoxicillin dual therapy versus bismuth-containing quadruple therapy for *Helicobacter pylori* eradication: A systematic review and meta-analysis. Helicobacter. 2024;**29**(1): e13040

[5] Chey WD, Mégraud F, Laine L, López LJ, Hunt BJ, Howden CW. Vonoprazan triple and dual therapy for *Helicobacter pylori* infection in the United States and Europe: Randomized clinical trial. Gastroenterology. 2022; **163**(3):608-619

[6] Graham DY. Why the Vonoprazan *Helicobacter pylori* therapies in the US-European trial produced unacceptable cure rates. Digestive Diseases and Sciences. 2023;**68**(5):1691-1697

[7] Xia H, Keane CT, Beattie S, O'Morain CA. Standardization of disk diffusion test and its clinical significance for susceptibility testing of metronidazole against *Helicobacter pylori*. Antimicrobial Agents and Chemotherapy. 1994;**38**(10):2357-2361

[8] Jearth V, Rath MM, Chatterjee A, Kale A, Panigrahi MK. Drug-resistant *Helicobacter pylori*: Diagnosis and evidence-based approach. Diagnostics (Basel, Switzerland). 2023;**13**(18):2944

[9] Tang X, Shen Y, Song X, Benghezal M, Marshall BJ, Tang H, et al. Reassessment of the broth microdilution method for susceptibility testing of *Helicobacter pylori*. The Journal of Infectious Diseases. 2022;**226**(Suppl. 5): S486-s492

[10] Kotilea K, Iliadis E, Nguyen J, Salame A, Mahler T, Miendje Deyi VY, et al. Antibiotic resistance, heteroresistance, and eradication success of *Helicobacter pylori* infection in children. Helicobacter. 2023;**28**(5): e13006

[11] Nguyen TC, Le GKN, Pham DTH, Pham BV, Nguyen LTH, Che TH, et al. Antibiotic resistance and heteroresistance in *Helicobacter pylori* isolates from symptomatic Vietnamese children: A prospective multicenter study. Helicobacter. 2023;**28**(5):e13009

[12] Trespalacios AA, Rimbara E, Otero W, Reddy R, Graham DY. Improved allele-specific PCR assays for detection of clarithromycin and fluoroquinolone resistant of *Helicobacter pylori* in gastric biopsies: Identification of N87I mutation in GyrA. Diagnostic Microbiology and Infectious Disease. 2015;**81**(4):251-255

[13] Marrero, Rolon R, Cunningham SA, Mandrekar JN, Polo ET, Patel R. Clinical evaluation of a real-time PCR assay for simultaneous detection of *Helicobacter pylori* and genotypic markers of clarithromycin resistance directly from stool. Journal of Clinical Microbiology. 2021;**59**(5):e03040-20

[14] Li Y, Lv T, He C, Wang H, Cram DS, Zhou L, et al. Evaluation of multiplex ARMS-PCR for detection of *Helicobacter pylori* mutations conferring resistance to clarithromycin and levofloxacin. Gut Pathogens. 2020;**12**:35

[15] Binmaeil H, Hanafiah A, Mohamed Rose I, Raja Ali RA. Development and validation of multiplex quantitative PCR assay for detection of *Helicobacter pylori* and mutations conferring resistance to clarithromycin and levofloxacin in gastric biopsy. Infection and Drug Resistance. 2021;**14**:4129-4145

[16] Kim I, Maeng LS, Kim JS, Kim BW, Cheung DY, Kim JI, et al. Quantitative multiplex real-time polymerase chain reaction assay for the detection of *Helicobacter pylori* and clarithromycin resistance. BMC Microbiology. 2023; **23**(1):155

[17] Spiteri JA, Zahra G, Schembri J, Pisani A, Borg E, Spiteri N, et al. Identification of antibiotic resistance patterns in *Helicobacter pylori* strains isolated from gastric biopsies using real-time PCR and genotypic analysis. Annals of Gastroenterology. 2021;**34**(4):501-509

[18] Kovacheva-Slavova M, Valkov H, Angelov T, Tropcheva R, Vladimirov B. Screening for *Helicobacter pylori* infection and clarithromycin resistance using real-time polymerase chain reaction. European Review for Medical and Pharmacological Sciences. 2021; **25**(15):5042-5046

[19] Noh JH, Ahn JY, Choi J, Park YS, Na HK, Lee JH, et al. Real-time polymerase chain reaction for the detection of *Helicobacter pylori* and clarithromycin resistance. Gut and Liver. 2023;**17**(3):375-381

[20] Karmakar BC, Paul S, Basak S, Ghosh M, Mukherjee P, Das R, et al. Development and evaluation of a simple PCR assay and nested PCR for rapid detection of clarithromycin-resistant *Helicobacter pylori* from culture and directly from the biopsy samples in India. Gut Pathogens. 2023;**15**(1):7

[21] Xia H, Daw MA, Sant S, Beattie S, Keane CT, O'Morain CA. Clinical efficacy of triple therapy in *Helicobacter pylori*-associated duodenal ulcer. European Journal of Gastroenterology & Hepatology. 1993;**5**(3):141-144

[22] Buckley MJ, Xia HX, Hyde DM, Keane CT, O'Morain CA. Metronidazole resistance reduces efficacy of triple therapy and leads to secondary clarithromycin resistance. Digestive Diseases and Sciences. 1997;**42**(10): 2111-2115

[23] Xia HX, Gilvarry J, Beattie S, Hamilton H, Keane CT, Sweeney EC, et al. Recrudescence of *Helicobacter pylori* infection in patients with healed duodenal ulcer after treatment with different regimens. The American Journal of Gastroenterology. 1995;**90**(8):1221-1225

[24] Wong WM, Gu Q, Wang WH, Fung FM, Berg DE, Lai KC, et al. Effects of primary metronidazole and clarithromycin resistance to *Helicobacter pylori* on omeprazole, metronidazole, and clarithromycin triple-therapy regimen in a region with high rates of metronidazole resistance. Clinical Infectious Diseases: An Official Publication of the Infectious Diseases Society of America. 2003;**37**(7):882-889

[25] Arenas A, Serrano C, Quiñones L, Harris P, Sandoval M, Lavanderos M, et al. High prevalence of clarithromycin resistance and effect on *Helicobacter pylori* eradication in a population from Santiago, Chile: Cohort study and meta-analysis. Scientific Reports. 2019;**9**(1): 20070

[26] An B, Moon BS, Kim H, Lim HC, Lee YC, Lee G, et al. Antibiotic resistance in *Helicobacter pylori* strains and its effect on *H. Pylori* eradication rates in a single center in Korea. Annals of Laboratory Medicine. 2013;**33**(6): 415-419

[27] Perna F, Zullo A, Ricci C, Hassan C, Morini S, Vaira D. Levofloxacin-based triple therapy for *Helicobacter pylori* re-treatment: Role of bacterial resistance. Digestive and Liver Disease: Official Journal of the Italian Society of Gastroenterology and the Italian Association for the Study of the Liver. 2007;**39**(11):1001-1005

[28] Lv ZF, Wang FC, Zheng HL, Wang B, Xie Y, Zhou XJ, et al. Meta-analysis: Is combination of tetracycline and amoxicillin suitable for *Helicobacter pylori* infection? World Journal of Gastroenterology. 2015;**21**(8):2522-2533

[29] Li M, Wang X, Meng W, Dai Y, Wang W. Empirical versus tailored therapy based on genotypic resistance detection for *Helicobacter pylori* eradication: A systematic review and meta-analysis. Therapeutic Advances in Gastroenterology. 2023;**16**: 17562848231196357

[30] Glupczynski Y, Mégraud F, Lopez-Brea M, Andersen LP. European multicentre survey of in vitro antimicrobial resistance in *Helicobacter pylori*. European Journal of Clinical Microbiology & Infectious Diseases: Official Publication of the European Society of Clinical Microbiology. 2001; **20**(11):820-823

[31] Tang X, Wang Z, Shen Y, Song X, Benghezal M, Marshall BJ, et al. Antibiotic resistance patterns of *Helicobacter pylori* strains isolated from the Tibet autonomous region, China. BMC Microbiology. 2022;**22**(1):196

[32] Li J, Deng J, Wang Z, Li H, Wan C. Antibiotic resistance of *Helicobacter pylori* strains isolated from pediatric patients in Southwest China. Frontiers in Microbiology. 2020;**11**:621791

[33] Kuo CJ, Lee CH, Chang ML, Lin CY, Lin WR, Su MY, et al. Multidrug resistance: The clinical dilemma of refractory *Helicobacter pylori* infection. Journal of Microbiology, Immunology, and Infection = Wei Mian Yu Gan Ran Za Zhi. 2021;**54**(6):1184-1187

[34] The European Committee on Antimicrobial Susceptibility Testing. Breakpoint tables for interpretation of MICs and zone diameters.Version 12.0. 2022 [Accessed: March 1, 2024]. Available from: https://www.eucast.org/fileadmin/src/media/PDFs/EUCAST_files/Breakpoint_tables/v_12.0_Breakpoint_Tables.pdf

[35] Dore M, Cirks B, Gleeson T. Eradicating multi-drug-resistant *Helicobacter pylori* with four times daily lansoprazole. The American Journal of Medicine. 2016;**129**(4):e21-e22

[36] Xia HX, Buckley M, Keane CT, O'Morain CA. Clarithromycin resistance in *Helicobacter pylori*: Prevalence in untreated dyspeptic patients and stability in vitro. The Journal of Antimicrobial Chemotherapy. 1996; **37**(3):473-481

[37] Ogata SK, Gales AC, Kawakami E. Antimicrobial susceptibility testing for *Helicobacter pylori* isolates from Brazilian children and adolescents: Comparing agar dilution, E-test, and disk diffusion. Brazilian Journal of Microbiology: [Publication of the Brazilian Society for Microbiology]. 2014;**45**(4):1439-1448

[38] Sánchez MA, Sánchez del Saz B, Loza E, Baquero F, Cantón R. Evaluation of the OSIRIS video reader system for

disk diffusion susceptibility test reading. Clinical Microbiology and Infection: The Official Publication of the European Society of Clinical Microbiology and Infectious Diseases. 2001;7(7):352-357

[39] Hombach M, Zbinden R, Böttger EC. Standardisation of disk diffusion results for antibiotic susceptibility testing using the sirscan automated zone reader. BMC Microbiology. 2013;**13**(1):225

[40] Argueta EA, Ho JJC, Elfanagely Y, D'Agata E, Moss SF. Clinical implication of drug resistance for *H. Pylori* management. Antibiotics (Basel, Switzerland). 2022;**11**(12):1684

[41] Ansari S, Yamaoka Y. *Helicobacter pylori* infection, its laboratory diagnosis, and antimicrobial resistance: A perspective of clinical relevance. Clinical Microbiology Reviews. 2022;**35**(3):e0025821

[42] Ding SZ, Du YQ, Lu H, Wang WH, Cheng H, Chen SY, et al. Chinese consensus report on family-based *Helicobacter pylori* infection control and management (2021 edition). Gut. 2022; **71**(2):238-253

[43] Tshibangu-Kabamba E, Yamaoka Y. *Helicobacter pylori* infection and antibiotic resistance - from biology to clinical implications. Nature Reviews Gastroenterology & Hepatology. 2021; **18**(9):613-629

[44] Ng HY, Leung WK, Cheung KS. Antibiotic resistance, susceptibility testing and stewardship in *Helicobacter pylori* infection. International Journal of Molecular Sciences. 2023;**24**(14):11708

[45] Versalovic J, Shortridge D, Kibler K, Griffy MV, Beyer J, Flamm RK, et al. Mutations in 23S rRNA are associated with clarithromycin resistance in *Helicobacter pylori*. Antimicrobial Agents and Chemotherapy. 1996;**40**(2):477-480

[46] Gong Y, Yuan Y. Resistance mechanisms of *Helicobacter pylori* and its dual target precise therapy. Critical Reviews in Microbiology. 2018;**44**(3): 371-392

[47] Dailidiene D, Bertoli MT, Miciuleviciene J, Mukhopadhyay AK, Dailide G, Pascasio MA, et al. Emergence of tetracycline resistance in *Helicobacter pylori*: Multiple mutational changes in 16S ribosomal DNA and other genetic loci. Antimicrobial Agents and Chemotherapy. 2002;**46**(12):3940-3946

[48] Gerrits MM, de Zoete MR, Arents NL, Kuipers EJ, Kusters JG. 16S rRNA mutation-mediated tetracycline resistance in *Helicobacter pylori*. Antimicrobial Agents and Chemotherapy. 2002;**46**(9):2996-3000

[49] Trieber CA, Taylor DE. Mutations in the 16S rRNA genes of *Helicobacter pylori* mediate resistance to tetracycline. Journal of Bacteriology. 2002;**184**(8): 2131-2140

[50] Gerrits MM, Godoy AP, Kuipers EJ, Ribeiro ML, Stoof J, Mendonça S, et al. Multiple mutations in or adjacent to the conserved penicillin-binding protein motifs of the penicillin-binding protein 1A confer amoxicillin resistance to *Helicobacter pylori*. Helicobacter. 2006; **11**(3):181-187

[51] Okamoto T, Yoshiyama H, Nakazawa T, Park ID, Chang MW, Yanai H, et al. A change in PBP1 is involved in amoxicillin resistance of clinical isolates of *Helicobacter pylori*. The Journal of Antimicrobial Chemotherapy. 2002;**50**(6):849-856

[52] Garcia M, Raymond J, Garnier M, Cremniter J, Burucoa C. Distribution of spontaneous gyrA mutations in 97 fluoroquinolone-resistant *Helicobacter*

pylori isolates collected in France. Antimicrobial Agents and Chemotherapy. 2012;**56**(1):550-551

[53] Nishizawa T, Suzuki H. Mechanisms of *Helicobacter pylori* antibiotic resistance and molecular testing. Frontiers in Molecular Biosciences. 2014;**1**:19

[54] Boyanova L, Markovska R, Hadzhiyski P, Kandilarov N, Mitov I. Rifamycin use for treatment of *Helicobacter pylori* infection: A review of recent data. Future Microbiology. 2020; **15**:1185-1196

[55] Hays C, Burucoa C, Lehours P, Tran CT, Leleu A, Raymond J. Molecular characterization of *Helicobacter pylori* resistance to rifamycins. Helicobacter. 2018;**23**(1):e12451

[56] Beckman E, Saracino I, Fiorini G, Clark C, Slepnev V, Patel D, et al. A novel stool PCR test for *Helicobacter pylori* may predict clarithromycin resistance and eradication of infection at a high rate. Journal of Clinical Microbiology. 2017;**55**(8):2400-2405

[57] Lottspeich C, Schwarzer A, Panthel K, Koletzko S, Rüssmann H. Evaluation of the novel *Helicobacter pylori* ClariRes real-time PCR assay for detection and clarithromycin susceptibility testing of *H. Pylori* in stool specimens from symptomatic children. Journal of Clinical Microbiology. 2007; **45**(6):1718-1722

[58] Vécsei A, Innerhofer A, Binder C, Gizci H, Hammer K, Bruckdorfer A, et al. Stool polymerase chain reaction for *Helicobacter pylori* detection and clarithromycin susceptibility testing in children. Clinical Gastroenterology and Hepatology: The Official Clinical Practice Journal of the American Gastroenterological Association. 2010; **8**(3):309-312

[59] Scaletsky IC, Aranda KR, Garcia GT, Gonçalves ME, Cardoso SR, Iriya K, et al. Application of real-time PCR stool assay for *Helicobacter pylori* detection and clarithromycin susceptibility testing in Brazilian children. Helicobacter. 2011; **16**(4):311-315

[60] Redondo JJ, Keller PM, Zbinden R, Wagner K. A novel RT-PCR for the detection of *Helicobacter pylori* and identification of clarithromycin resistance mediated by mutations in the 23S rRNA gene. Diagnostic Microbiology and Infectious Disease. 2018;**90**(1):1-6

[61] Schabereiter-Gurtner C, Hirschl AM, Dragosics B, Hufnagl P, Puz S, Kovách Z, et al. Novel real-time PCR assay for detection of *Helicobacter pylori* infection and simultaneous clarithromycin susceptibility testing of stool and biopsy specimens. Journal of Clinical Microbiology. 2004;**42**(10):4512-4518

[62] Sun L, Talarico S, Yao L, He L, Self S, You Y, et al. Droplet digital PCR-based detection of clarithromycin resistance in *Helicobacter pylori* isolates reveals frequent Heteroresistance. Journal of Clinical Microbiology. 2018;**56**(9): e00019-18

[63] Saracino IM, Pavoni M, Zullo A, Fiorini G, Lazzarotto T, Borghi C, et al. Next generation sequencing for the prediction of the antibiotic resistance in *Helicobacter pylori*: A literature review. Antibiotics (Basel, Switzerland). 2021; **10**(4):437

[64] Fernández-Caso B, Miqueleiz A, Alarcón T. Whole genome sequencing for studying *Helicobacter pylori* antimicrobial resistance. Antibiotics (Basel, Switzerland). 2023;**12**(7):1135

[65] Hu L, Zeng X, Ai Q, Liu C, Zhang X, Chen Y, et al. Long-read- and short-read-based whole-genome sequencing reveals the antibiotic resistance pattern of *Helicobacter pylori*. Microbiology Spectrum. 2023;**11**(3): e0452222

[66] Zhou Y, Zhong Z, Hu S, Wang J, Deng Y, Li X, et al. A survey of *Helicobacter pylori* antibiotic-resistant genotypes and strain lineages by whole-genome sequencing in China. Antimicrobial Agents and Chemotherapy. 2022;**66**(6):e0218821

[67] Fauzia KA, Alfaray RI, Yamaoka Y. Advantages of whole genome sequencing in mitigating the *Helicobacter pylori* antimicrobial resistance problem. Microorganisms. 2023;**11**(5):1239

[68] Lauener FN, Imkamp F, Lehours P, Buissonnière A, Benejat L, Zbinden R, et al. Genetic determinants and prediction of antibiotic resistance phenotypes in *Helicobacter pylori*. Journal of Clinical Medicine. 2019;**8**(1):53

[69] Hulten KG, Genta RM, Kalfus IN, Zhou Y, Zhang H, Graham DY. Comparison of culture with Antibiogram to next-generation sequencing using bacterial isolates and formalin-fixed. Paraffin-Embedded Gastric Biopsies. Gastroenterology. 2021;**161**(5): 1433-1442.e1432

[70] Yin G, Bie S, Gu H, Shu X, Zheng W, Peng K, et al. Application of gene chip technology in the diagnostic and drug resistance detection of *Helicobacter pylori* in children. Journal of Gastroenterology and Hepatology. 2020; **35**(8):1331-1339

[71] Beaulaurier J, Zhang XS, Zhu S, Sebra R, Rosenbluh C, Deikus G, et al. Single molecule-level detection and long read-based phasing of epigenetic variations in bacterial methylomes. Nature Communications. 2015;**6**:7438

[72] Satam H, Joshi K, Mangrolia U, Waghoo S, Zaidi G, Rawool S, et al. Next-generation sequencing technology: Current trends and advancements. Biology. 2023;**12**(7):997

[73] Kocsmár É, Kocsmár I, Buzás GM, Szirtes I, Wacha J, Takáts A, et al. *Helicobacter pylori* heteroresistance to clarithromycin in adults-new data by in situ detection and improved concept. Helicobacter. 2020;**25**(1):e12670

[74] Kim JJE, Kocsmár I, Buzás GM, Szirtes I, Rusz O, Diczházi C, et al. Efficacy of clarithromycin depends on the bacterial density in clarithromycin-heteroresistant *Helicobacter pylori* infections: An In situ detected susceptibility and quantitative morphometry-based retrospective study. Pathology Oncology Research: POR. 2021;**27**:1609863

[75] Xia HY, Keane CT, O'Morain CA. Eradication rate of *Helicobcter pylori*. Gut. 1995;**37**(4):591-592

[76] Arévalo-Jaimes BV, Rojas-Rengifo DF, Jaramillo CA, de Molano BM, Vera-Chamorro JF, Del Pilar DM. Genotypic determination of resistance and heteroresistance to clarithromycin in *Helicobacter pylori* isolates from antrum and corpus of Colombian symptomatic patients. BMC Infectious Diseases. 2019; **19**(1):546

[77] Kakiuchi T. Accurate evaluation of pediatric *Helicobacter pylori* heteroresistance contributes to further improving the quality of tailored therapy. Pediatric Research. 2024. DOI: 10.1038/s41390-024-03072-z [Online ahead of print]

[78] Matsuda K. PCR-based detection methods for single-nucleotide polymorphism or mutation: Real-time PCR and its substantial contribution toward technological refinement. Advances in Clinical Chemistry. 2017;**80**: 45-72

[79] Chen MJ, Chen PY, Fang YJ, Bair MJ, Chen CC, Chen CC, et al. Molecular testing-guided therapy versus susceptibility testing-guided therapy in first-line and third-line *Helicobacter pylori* eradication: Two multicentre, open-label, randomised controlled, non-inferiority trials. The Lancet Gastroenterology & Hepatology. 2023; **8**(7):623-634

[80] Li CL, Zhou K, Zhang YX, Suo BJ, Tian XL, Zhang YX, et al. Tailored therapy guided by genotypic resistance of clarithromycin and levofloxacin detected by polymerase chain reaction in the first-line treatment of *Helicobacter pylori* infection. Journal of Digestive Diseases. 2024;**25**(1):36-43

[81] Lin K, Huang L, Wang Y, Li K, Ye Y, Yang S, et al. Efficacy of genotypic susceptibility-guided tailored therapy for *Helicobacter pylori* infection: A systematic review and single arm meta-analysis. Helicobacter. 2023;**28**(6): e13015

[82] Han X, Yu X, Gao X, Wang X, Tay CY, Wei X, et al. Quantitative PCR of string-test collected gastric material: A feasible approach to detect *Helicobacter pylori* and its resistance against clarithromycin and levofloxacin for susceptibility-guided therapy. Helicobacter. 2023;**28**(4):e12985

[83] Wang L, Li Z, Tay CY, Marshall BJ, Gu B. Multicentre, cross-sectional surveillance of *Helicobacter pylori* prevalence and antibiotic resistance to clarithromycin and levofloxacin in urban China using the string test coupled with quantitative PCR. The Lancet. Microbe. 2024. DOI: 10.1016/S2666-5247(24) 00027-2 [Online ahead of print]

[84] Wang L, Lai JX, Si YT, Cui XX, Umar Z, Ru XJ, et al. Quantitative polymerase chain reaction (qPCR)-based rapid diagnosis of *Helicobacter pylori* infection and antibiotic resistance. Journal of Visualized Experiments: JoVE. 2023;**197**:e65689

[85] Tang JW, Li F, Liu X, Wang JT, Xiong XS, Lu XY, et al. Detection of *Helicobacter pylori* infection in human gastric fluid through surface-enhanced Raman spectroscopy coupled with machine learning algorithms. Laboratory Investigation; A Journal of Technical Methods and Pathology. 2024;**104**(2): 100310

[86] Malfertheiner P, Megraud F, Rokkas T, Gisbert JP, Liou JM, Schulz C, et al. Management of *Helicobacter pylori* infection: The Maastricht VI/Florence consensus report. Gut. 2022:1724-1762

[87] Du RC, Hu YX, Ouyang Y, Ling LX, Xu JY, Sa R, et al. Vonoprazan and amoxicillin dual therapy as the first-line treatment of *Helicobacter pylori* infection: A systematic review and meta-analysis. Helicobacter. 2024;**29**(1):e13039

[88] Liu T, Chai S, Li M, Chen X, Xie Y, Zhao Z, et al. A nanoparticle-based sonodynamic therapy reduces *Helicobacter pylori* infection in mouse without disrupting gut microbiota. Nature Communications. 2024;**15**(1):844

Chapter 2

Interleukin 17 and Interferon-Gamma, Key Cytokines for Inflammation and Diagnosis in *Helicobacter pylori* and Gastric Malignancies

Mario M. D'Elios and Chiara Della Bella

Abstract

Helicobacter pylori infection is characterized by an inflammatory infiltrate that might be an important antecedent of gastric cancer. Interferon-gamma (IFN-γ) and interleukin (IL)-17 are key cytokines produced by gastric T cells in *Helicobacter pylori*-infected patients with gastric malignancies. We studied the levels of serum IL-17A in subjects positive to *Helicobacter pylori* infection and diagnosed with gastric intestinal metaplasia and dysplasia, as well as in patients with *Helicobacter pylori* infection and non-atrophic gastritis, along with control subjects. Results showed that *Helicobacter pylori* can cause inflammation in the stomach, specifically in cases of gastric intestinal metaplasia and dysplasia in infected patients, leading to a significant rise in IL-17A serum levels. Accordingly, we propose to consider measuring serum IL-17A for managing *Helicobacter pylori*-infected patients, and potentially for predicting the risk of developing gastric cancer.

Keywords: *Helicobacter pylori*, gastric cancer, gastric inflammation, interleukin 17, interferon-gamma, serum cytokine, T cells

1. Introduction

Helicobacter pylori (*H. pylori*) is a spiral, microaerophilic, Gram-negative bacterium. *H. pylori* infection is one of the most common bacterial infections that afflicts over 50% of the world's population and leads to persistent infections in the stomach throughout a person's life. The bacterium is the major contributor to several gastric diseases, including gastric adenocarcinoma, autoimmune gastritis, gastric mucosa-associated lymphoid tissue (MALT) lymphoma, gastric autoimmunity, and peptic ulcer [1–11]. The World Health Organization classifies *H. pylori* as an IARC class I carcinogen that is the dominant risk factor for distal gastric cancer [12]. Eradicating *H. pylori* has been shown to decline the incidence of gastric cancer [13–16]. The presence of *H. pylori* infection in the stomach triggers a complex and multiform inflammation characterized by the infiltration of immune cells and the local production of various inflammatory mediators, including cytokines and chemokines [17]. The host's immune system can either fight the *H. pylori* infection or the bacterium can evade the host's defense mechanisms; in the latter case, the chronic infection can lead to the development of gastric cancer [18]. Certain factors of *H. pylori*, such as the cytotoxin VacA and gamma-glutamyl transpeptidase GGT, can suppress the immune system and impair both innate and acquired immunity. These factors exert their influence on antigen-presenting cells and T cells [19–22]. Once in the stomach, *H. pylori* first activates the innate immunity, recruiting macrophages and neutrophils which initiate and sustain the inflammatory cascade. The gastric epithelium reacts to the bacterium; the resident macrophages are activated by Toll-like receptors (TLR) with bacterial products such as LPS, CagA, VacA, HP0175, heat shock proteins such as HP-NAP [23, 24]. Furthermore, *H. pylori* peptidoglycan may result in activation of the NOD-1 receptors. These stimuli cause a massive release of chemokines such as IL-8, a strong activator for neutrophils, and inflammatory cytokines such as IL-1, IL-6, TNF-α, IFN-α, IL-12, and IL-23. In particular, IL-12 and IL-23 secreted by both macrophages and neutrophils, play a key role in natural host defense and are decisive in driving the subsequent adoptive cell response polarized as Th1. [25, 26].

Studies about host immune responses to *H. pylori* infection have mainly focused on Th1, Th17, and Th2 cells. Some *H. pylori* strains may be more virulent than others, and the involved immune responses may depend on the type of the host immune response. A large body of clinical and experimental evidence has demonstrated that *H. pylori* at any stage of the infection activates the production of high levels of IFN-γ. On the one hand, IFN-γ is necessary for the control of infection; on the other hand, whether its production is abnormally maintained for a very long period might lead to gastric immunopathology and eventually to gastric cancer [27–30]. In *H. pylori* infection, the adoptive immunity is predominantly mediated by Th1 and Th17 cells. In patients with gastric precancerous lesions and gastric adenocarcinoma, high gastric IL-17 secretion is associated with IFN-γ production [2, 23, 29, 31–33].

Mice with *H. pylori* infection may exhibit a dual Th17/Th1 response, with a first Th17 action followed by the Th1 response. Mice treated with anti-IL-17 antibody showed a notable decrease in *H. pylori* burden and stomach inflammation, unlike those treated with a control antibody. IL-17(−/−) mice exhibited decreased *H. pylori* colonization and reduced gastric inflammation as well [34]. The precise mechanisms underlying Th17 involvement in gastric tumorigenesis are yet to be established. However, Kang JH et al. in their study suggest that IL-17A promotes gastric carcinogenesis, in part, by regulating IL-17RC/NF-κB/NOX1 pathway [35]. Furthermore, *H. pylori* CagY protein mainly induces the production of IFN-γ and IL-17 by T helper lymphocytes in the stomach, enhancing B cell growth and potentially causing gastric MALT lymphoma. The increased production of IL-17 is associated with more severe forms of *H. pylori*-associated diseases, especially with gastric premalignant and malignant lesions [29, 36].

The severity of symptoms caused by *H. pylori* infection is related to the predominant subset of T cell-mediated immune response that subsequently occurs. It has been shown that in the infected gastric mucosa, a specific pro-inflammatory response to *H. pylori*, Th1 polarization, correlates with more severe disease progression. Moreover, in uncomplicated chronic gastritis (UCG), an *H. pylori*-specific T component Th1/Th2 mixed was found to prevail [27, 37–43].

In the gastric mucosa infected with *H. pylori*, the signaling pathway for Th1 is stimulated by IL-12 [44]. A local Th0 response, including interleukin-4 production by

Th2 cells, represents an individual host factor that contributes to lowering the degree of gastric inflammation and preventing ulcer complications. Thus, in uncomplicated chronic gastritis, the Th1 response is balanced by a concomitant Th2 response [27]. The immune profile in the reaction to *H. pylori* infection can be modulated by co-infections (helminth parasitism and "African enigma") or comorbidities. Some population surveys have shown an inverse association between *H. pylori* infection and Th2-related pathology like atopy, allergy, and asthma [45–48]. The pathogenic potential of polarized Th1 responses in *H. pylori* infection finds indirect support in the phenomenon commonly known as "the African enigma" by which the high prevalence of *H. pylori* infection in Africa is not supported by a correlated high incidence of peptic ulcer disease and gastric cancer [49, 50]. One possible explanation for this phenomenon is the simultaneous presence of an endemic high parasitic burden, which is known to trigger a Th2-like immune response. The Th2 polarization stimulated by helminth infections could attenuate the Th1-like immune response induced by *H. pylori* infection and, consequently, the gastro-duodenal pathology induced by the bacteria. This hypothesis has been supported by experimental studies in which co-infection of mice with *Helicobacter felis* and a natural murine helminth (*Heligmosomoides polygyrus*) led to a reduction in Th1-mediated gastric atrophy, which is considered a pre-malignant lesion [51]. These Th2 responses may serve to protect individuals with *H. pylori* infection from developing peptic ulcers and gastric cancer.

Inflammatory cytokines and chemokines can trigger several injurious effects on gastric epithelial cells, including uncontrolled proliferation, resistance to apoptosis, and DNA damage. These deleterious effects can eventually culminate in the cancerous transformation of the gastric cells [52–54]. The carcinogenic pathway leading to gastric cancer, which is closely associated with inflammation, is a multi-step process that takes place in nearly 1% of individuals affected by chronic *H. pylori* infection. It is important to note that while non-atrophic gastritis (NAG) develops in almost all patients infected with *H. pylori*, in some cases the inflammation progresses to more advanced stages of pre-malignancy, such as gastric intestinal metaplasia (IM) and dysplasia (DYS) of the stomach [55, 56]. In the later stages of this inflammation-induced carcinogenic process, various types of genetic instabilities occur, characterized by diverse and potentially harmful clonal assemblies [44, 57–60]. In this chapter, we will review the different types of inflammation going on in the stomach of patients with *H. pylori* infection and different clinical outcomes as gastric autoimmunity, gastric MALT lymphoma and we will focus especially on gastric adenocarcinoma and gastric premalignant lesions, such as gastric intestinal metaplasia and gastric dysplasia, as well as on the potential usefulness of interleukin 17A (IL-17A) for the management of patients with *H. pylori* infection and gastric adenocarcinoma or gastric pre-malignancies.

2. *Helicobacter pylori* and gastric autoimmunity

H. pylori infection is closely linked to gastric autoimmunity. Numerous clinical and epidemiological studies suggest that a significant majority of patients with autoimmune gastritis (AIG) either currently have or have had *H. pylori* infection [10]. AIG is a chronic inflammatory disease characterized by autoimmune-mediated destruction of parietal and zymogenic cells of the corpus and fundus of the stomach which leads to atrophy of the gastric corpus mucosa. Pernicious anemia (PA) may develop in advanced AIG, due to the lack of Intrinsic factor (IF) and related cobalamin decrease [61]. Remarkable resemblances can be highlighted between classical AIG and *H. pylori*-induced corpus atrophic gastritis [62]; moreover, the AIG preclinical stages can be effectively regressed by eradication of the bacteria [63–65]. *H. pylori* prompts the production of autoantibodies targeting gastric mucosal protein epitopes in about half of infected individuals [56–70]. The process of molecular mimicry underlying the induction of autoimmunity in AIG takes place against the gastric pump H^+/K^+ ATPase antigen, the proton pump located in the secretory canaliculi of the parietal cells [71]. The H^+/K^+ ATPase is the primary autoantigen responsible for the immunopathology in autoimmune gastritis (AIG) [72]. In mice, unlike what happens in humans, gastric autoantibody production due to *H. pylori* infection is caused by a mimicry process with LPS Lewis blood-group antigens and Lewis antigens on the glycosylated α-subunit [62, 63, 73].

In humans with AIG, *H. pylori* infection activates gastric T cells, a significant proportion of which exhibit cross-reactivity against both *H. pylori* peptide antigens

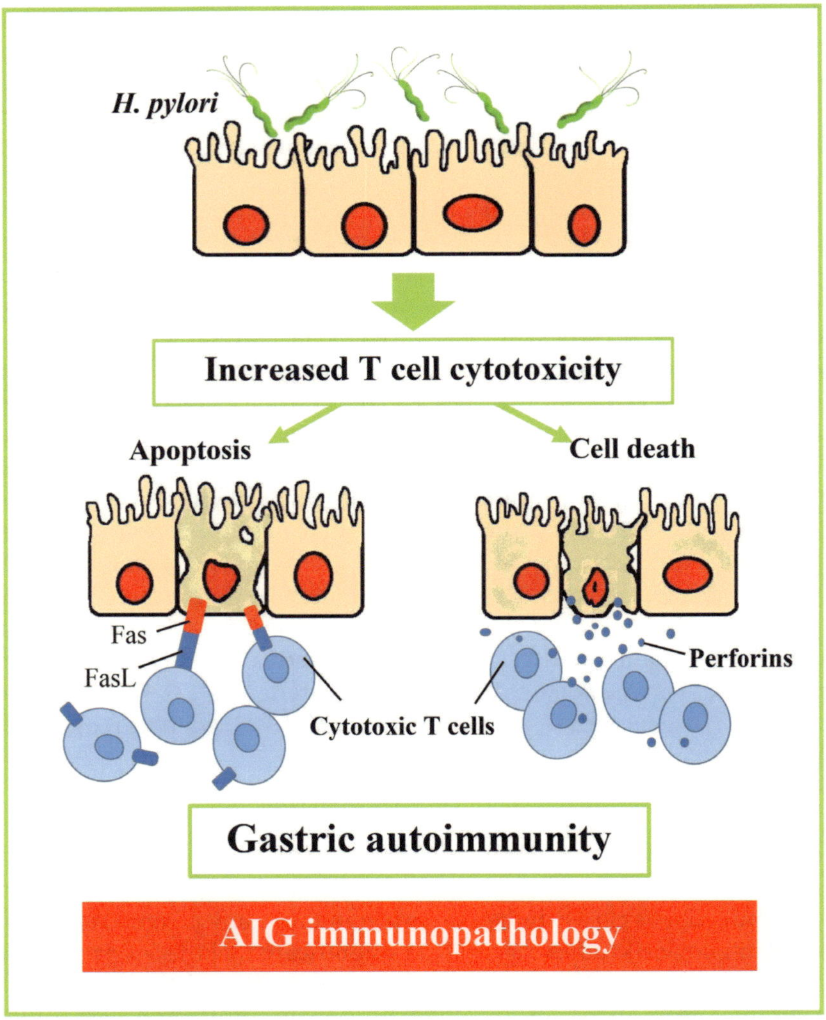

Figure 1.
Immunopathogenesis of autoimmune gastritis (AIG).

and H^+/K^+ ATPase through a mechanism involving molecular mimicry [10, 74]. The identification of these *H. pylori*/ATPase-specific T cells explains the correlation between *H. pylori* infection and corpus atrophic gastritis. The research by Bergman et al. aimed to determine the epitopes of the human gastric ATPase α and β chains recognized by the autoreactive T cell clones infiltrating gastric biopsies of AIG subjects. Their data identified a group of the H^+/K^+ ATPase autoantigens that resulted the same in all the enrolled AIG subjects, regardless of *H. pylori* infection status [75, 76]. Interestingly, these bacterial crossreactive immunogenic antigens were not constituent of the established immunodominant proteins *of H. pylori* CagA, VacA and Urease, at the base of peptic ulcer [37] and chronic antral gastritis etiopathogenesis [27]. Rather, these *H. pylori* cross-reactive epitopes mainly are codified by the bacteria housekeeping genes and are HLA-DR-restricted [74]. When stimulated with their specific cross-reactive bacterial peptide, all the ATPase/*H. pylori*-specific T cell clones obtained by gastric mucosa of AIG patients exhibited a Th1 phenotype, with a cytokine milieu composed of high amount of IFN-γ, without IL-4 and IL-5 secretion [74–76]. Following activation, all the aforementioned ATPase/*H. pylori*-specific T cell clones showed cytotoxic activity by Fas-Fas ligand (FasL)-mediated apoptosis or by perforin-mediated cytotoxicity against gastric epithelial cells [55] which, following the action of IFN-γ and TNF-α, showed a heightened receptor Fas on their membrane [77], contributing to their apoptosis induction (**Figure 1**) [78]. Consequently, in certain patients, likely influenced by unknown genetic or environmental factors, *H. pylori* infection causes an excessive cellular immune response at the gastric level, leading to gastric autoimmunity through a mechanism of molecular mimicry.

3. *Helicobacter pylori* and gastric MALT lymphoma

Extranodal marginal zone B cell lymphoma of mucosa-associated lymphoid tissue (MALT lymphoma) is the third most common type of non-Hodgkin lymphoma [79, 80]. The stomach has the highest incidence of MALT lymphoma, with typical clinical and histopathologic features [81]. The association between *H. pylori* infection and gastric MALT lymphoma has been established through the finding of the bacteria into a large number of MALT lymphoma biopsies [82]. *H. pylori*-related low-grade gastric MALT lymphoma serves as a model for studying the interplay between chronic infection, immune response, and lymphomagenesis. This tumor is notable as the first neoplasia that could be totally cured in early stages, thanks to the removal of *H. pylori* infection by antibiotic therapy [7]. The establishment of low-grade B cell gastric MALT lymphoma is due to *H. pylori* infection in the presence of *H. pylori*-specific T cells that provide an uncontrolled help function on tumor cell proliferation. Tumor cells are memory B cells that remain responsive to differentiation signals, such as CD40 costimulation and cytokines produced by bacterial-specific Th cells. Thus, the proliferation of B lymphocytes is strictly dependent on *H. pylori*-specific T helper lymphocytes [83–85].

In the early phases, this tumor is responsive to the withdrawal of *H. pylori*-induced T cell help, describing the tumor's inclination to stay in its original location and its clinical resolution following the antibiotic therapy to remove the bacterium. Examining the helper function given by gastric *H. pylori*-specific T cell clones to B cells has revealed in-depth knowledge on the molecular and cellular processes linked to the development of low-grade gastric MALToma. The T helper cells isolated and amplified by cloning were tested for their antigen specificity for *H. pylori*, achieving a positivity of 3–20%. The majority of the T cell clones obtained was not specific for the well-known proteins CagA, VacA, Urease or HSP. Each *H. pylori*-specific T helper clone obtained *in vitro* from gastric MALToma infiltrate produced IL-2 and a milieu of B cell-activating cytokines, such as IL-4 and IL-13. These clones, after activation with the specific bacterial antigens showed a potent help function for B cell activation and proliferation. B cells in MALToma patients proliferate when exposed to *H. pylori*, but the B cell growth stimulated by bacterial antigens requires T helper cells to occur [86].

Recently, we could demonstrate that CagY is an important *H. pylori* antigen and is able to drive mucosal activation and B cell proliferation in gastric low-grade MALT lymphoma [36]. In patients with chronic gastritis, whether with or without ulcers, the helper function toward B cells exerted by *H. pylori* antigen-stimulated gastric T cell clones was negatively regulated by the concurrent cytolytic killing of B cells [27, 37]. Conversely, gastric T cell clones from MALToma were incapable of downmodulating their antigen-induced help for B cell proliferation. The perforine-mediated cytotoxic function of these T cell clones against autologous B lymphocytes was absent. The Fas-FasL mediated apoptosis toward tumor cells was founded in a small number of *H. pylori*-specific T helper clones from MALT lymphoma in comparison to the ones obtained from the mucosa of patients with uncomplicated chronic gastritis. The dysfunction of perforin-mediated cytotoxicity and the restricted capacity to induce Fas-FasL mediated apoptosis were unique to T cells that infiltrated MALTomas. T helper lymphocytes specific for *H. pylori* antigens obtained from the peripheral blood of the same subjects exhibited similar cytolytic potential and proapoptotic activity as T helper cells from patients with chronic gastritis [86]. Mice with cytotoxic T cells deficient in perforin, develop lymphomas with age [87, 88] and, more frequently and earlier, B cell lymphoma occurs in mice lacking both perforin and beta-2 microglobulin (β2m). Furthermore, B cell lymphomas originating from mice lacking both perforin and β2m are rejected by either NK cells or γδ T cells upon transplantation into WT mice, rather than by αβ T cells (as observed in tumors from mice lacking only perforin), emphasizing that the tumor cell's membrane expression of MHC class I molecules is important in deciding which effector cell provide immune protection [89].

Interestingly, subgroups of lymphoma patients have been found to have mutations in the gene that codes for perforin [90], although, the involvement of this mutation in etiogenesis remains unclear. Mice lacking in the pro-apoptotic cytokine TNF-related apoptosis-inducing ligand (TRAIL) or with a mutate form of the death-inducing protein FasL have also been found to be vulnerable to developing late-onset spontaneous lymphomas [75, 76]. These research unequivocally underscore the important function of cytotoxic mechanisms in immune system regulation and/or suppression of natural tumor growth in mice. It is not clear why gastric T cells of MALToma lack mechanisms to control B cell growth despite providing potent support to B cells. VacA toxin has been shown to block the processing of antigens in antigen-presenting cells (APCs) and T cells, while it does not affect the release of perforin by NK cells [19, 21]. We can hypothesize that in some *H. pylori*-infected subjects, certain bacterial components can affect the regulatory cytotoxic mechanisms in gastric T cells that control B cell proliferation, thereby allowing exhaustive and unbalanced B cell help and lymphomagenesis to occur (**Figure 2**) [86, 91, 92].

DOI: http://dx.doi.org/10.5772/intechopen.1005301

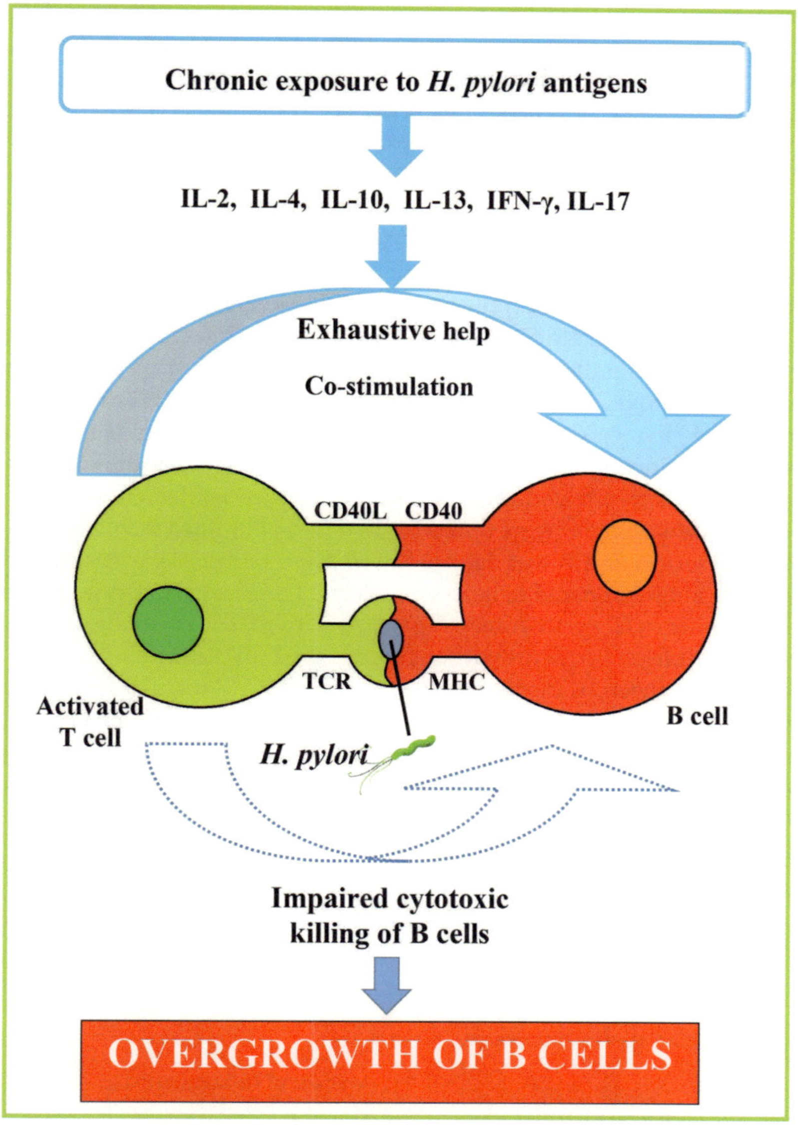

Figure 2.
Immunopathogenesis of gastric MALT lymphoma.

4. *Helicobacter pylori* and gastric pre-malignancies

A long-lasting gastric inflammation is considered risky for the development of gastric adenocarcinoma [93]. TNF-α and IL-1β are key cytokines for the development of a gastric niche that favors the onset of gastric cancer [94–96]. The continuous secretion of cytokines in the stomach, characterized by a chronic pattern, has the potential to influence the progression of gastric cancer [54, 97–101]. *H. pylori* is capable of triggering an innate immune response abundant in IL-1β, IL-6, transforming growth factor (TGF)-β, and IL-23 which are able to steer a T cell response towards the Th17 phenotype [96, 102]. Th17 inflammatory responses are orchestrated by T helper

17 cells, which release IL-17 and play a pivotal role in initiating numerous inflammatory pathways within the gastric environment [72]. Elevated levels of IL-17 have been identified in gastric tissues of individuals with *H. pylori* infection [32, 34, 103].

We recently focused on the type of gastric T cell responses in *H. pylori*-infected patients with gastric pre-malignant lesions, such as intestinal metaplasia/dysplasia (IM/DYS), by defining the cytokine profile secreted by infiltrating gastric T cells [29]. ELISpot assay for IL-17 demonstrated that gastric-derived T helper cells from *H. pylori*-infected IM/DYS patients significantly produced IL-17A in response to *H. pylori* antigen compared to unstimulated conditions and non-*H. pylori* antigens (tetanus toxoid). No significant IL-4 secretion from the same T cell lines was detected by ELISA. From the T cell infiltrating the gastric mucosa of these *H. pylori*-infected IM/DYS patients, 242 T cell clones were obtained and characterized for their function and responsiveness to *H. pylori*. No cytotoxic T cell clone was specific for *H. pylori*; 12% of $CD4^+$ T cell clones proliferated in response to *H. pylori* antigens and all of them demonstrated IL-17 secretion by the entire population, with 11/29 clones producing both IFN-γ and IL-17. The sera from *H. pylori*-infected IM/DYS patients, *H. pylori*-infected patients without IM/DYS and healthy controls were tested for IL-17A by Luminex technology. A significant increase in serum IL-17A was detected in *H. pylori*-infected patients with gastric premalignant lesions compared to healthy subjects. The serum IL-17A levels were significantly higher in *H. pylori*-infected patients with gastric premalignant lesions than in *H. pylori*-infected patients without gastric premalignant lesions.

The gastric precancerous cascade by Correa et al. [55, 56] highlights the progressive changes in the gastric mucosa caused by *H. pylori* infection and leading to gastric adenocarcinoma. *H. pylori* infection induces both innate and adoptive immune responses. The amount of IL-17 and the percentage of *H. pylori*-specific T helper 17 cells are in

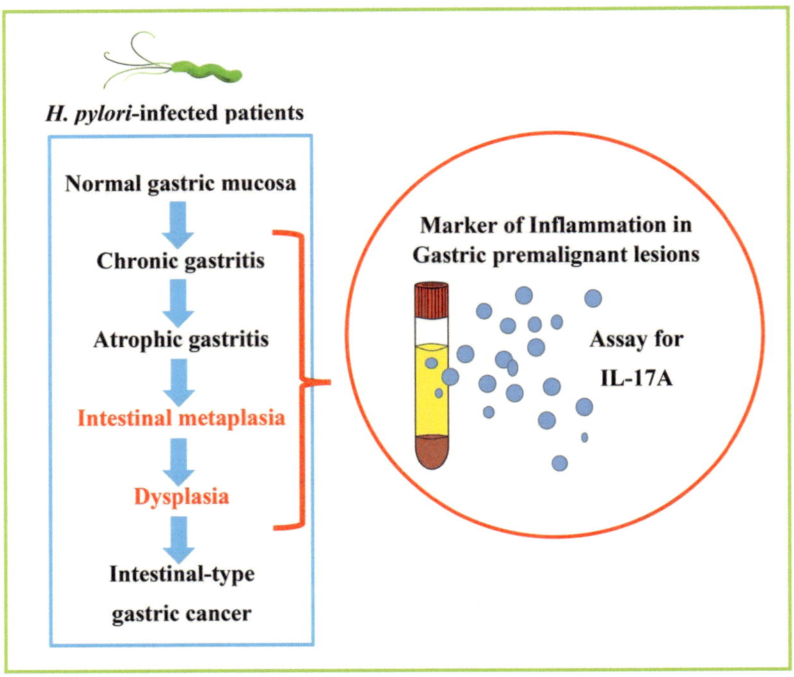

Figure 3.
IL-17A as a potential inflammatory marker for gastric cancer.

patients with gastric premalignant lesions and gastric adenocarcinoma significantly more elevated than the amount of IL-17 and Th17 cells found in patients with uncomplicated chronic gastritis. Thus, it is reasonable to hypothesize that the higher serum levels of IL-17 found in patients with gastric premalignant lesions are due to decades of higher activation of *H. pylori*-specific T helper 17 compartments in their gastric mucosa. Therefore, IL-17A plays a crucial role in causing inflammation in the gastric mucosa of patients with autoimmune atrophic gastritis without *H. pylori* infection [104], as well as being a key cytokine in the immunopathogenesis of gastric intestinal metaplasia and gastric dysplasia in *H. pylori*-infected patients, as shown in this study, both in the stomach and in the blood (**Figure 3**). As this study is a preliminary single-center research, it is crucial to conduct further multi-center inmvestigations on serum IL-17A levels in gastric adenocarcinoma to better understand the proposed test.

5. *Helicobacter pylori* and gastric adenocarcinoma

Gastric cancer remains a significant global public health challenge, ranking as the seventh most prevalent form of cancer worldwide and the fifth leading cause of cancer-related death, according to data from GLOBOCAN 2020. Globally, approximately 1.9 million individuals are currently diagnosed with gastric cancer, accounting for 3.6% of all cancer diagnoses. Furthermore, it stands as the fourth most common cause of cancer-related deaths on a global scale. These statistics underscore the ongoing importance of addressing gastric cancer as a major health concern [105]. It has been shown that there is a predominant T helper 17 and T helper 1 response in *H. pylori*-infected patients with gastric adenocarcinoma and in *H. pylori*-negative patients with autoimmune atrophic gastritis [33, 104, 106]. There were no clues on which *H. pylori* antigen was able to drive IL-17 production. It has been shown that the *H. pylori* HP0175 antigen can activate the inflammation of T cells in the stomach. T cell lines were obtained from Tumor-Infiltrating Lymphocyte (TIL) cells derived from the stomach of gastric adenocarcinoma patients and were tested for their IL-17 secretion after HP0175, TT, or PPD stimulation in ELISpot microplates. A significant proportion of all gastric-derived T cell lines specifically reacted to HP0175 by producing IL-17 in a dose-dependent manner, while non-*H. pylori* antigens like TT and PPD were ineffective at any concentration used.

Gastric biopsies obtained by *H. pylori*-infected patients showed an inflammatory infiltrate full of *H. pylori*-specific T cells actively producing IL-17. The IL-17 is produced by T cells following priming given by innate cells producing IL-23, TGF-β, etc. [23, 29, 31–33, 107, 108]. TILs were also characterized at the clonal level [101] for their HP0175 specificity, obtaining no $CD8^+$ clone significantly proliferated. In contrast, 7% of the $CD4^+$ T cell clones showed significant proliferation to HP0175. It is of note that *H. pylori* 0175 was able to induce the production by monocytes and neutrophils of several cytokines (IL-23, IL-1β, TGF-β, IL-6) known to have the ability to induce the production of IL-17 [23]. A similar study was carried out by testing the T cell response toward HP1454 in the gastric mucosa of *H. pylori*-positive patients with chronic gastritis and gastric adenocarcinoma [99]. T-cell blasts were recovered from gastric mucosa samples and cloned through limiting dilution. All $CD4^+$ and $CD8^+$ T cell clones obtained from gastric biopsies of *H. pylori*-positive subjects underwent testing for proliferation response to HP1454 in the presence of irradiated APCs. In uncomplicated chronic gastritis, 2.09% of the $CD4^+$ T cell clones were specific for HP1454, while in gastric adenocarcinoma 7.78% of the $CD4^+$ T cell clones exhibited significant proliferation to HP1454. Notably, none of the $CD8^+$ clones was specific for HP1454. Among the HP1454 specific T helper clones from uncomplicated chronic gastritis, 1/3 produced IFN-γ alone, 40% produced IL-17 alone, and 27% four produced both cytokines. Conversely, in gastric adenocarcinoma, upon stimulation with HP1454, 30% of HP1454-specific T cell clones produced IFN-γ alone, 23% produced IL-17 alone and 47% produced both IFN-γ and IL-17. Remarkably, HP1454-specific clones from the gastric mucosa of patients with gastric adenocarcinoma produced higher levels of tumor necrosis factor α and IL-17 compared to the HP1454-specific clones from patients with uncomplicated chronic gastritis. These findings collectively suggest that the protein HP1454, released by *H. pylori*-infected patients, plays a role in driving Th1 and Th17 inflammatory responses during chronic *H. pylori* infection and in patients with distal adenocarcinoma.

Sun et al. in a recent elegant study characterized in patients with gastric cancer the clonotype and trajectory analysis of gastric T cells by single-cell RNA-sequencing (scRNA-seq) [109]. They found that also $CD8^+$ T cells from gastric cancer patients produce IL-17 and promote tumor progression through IL-17, IL-22, and IL-26 signaling. IL-17 can, in turn, activate the STAT3 signaling pathway and promote epithelial-to-mesenchymal transition, migration, and invasiveness of gastric cancer cells [110].

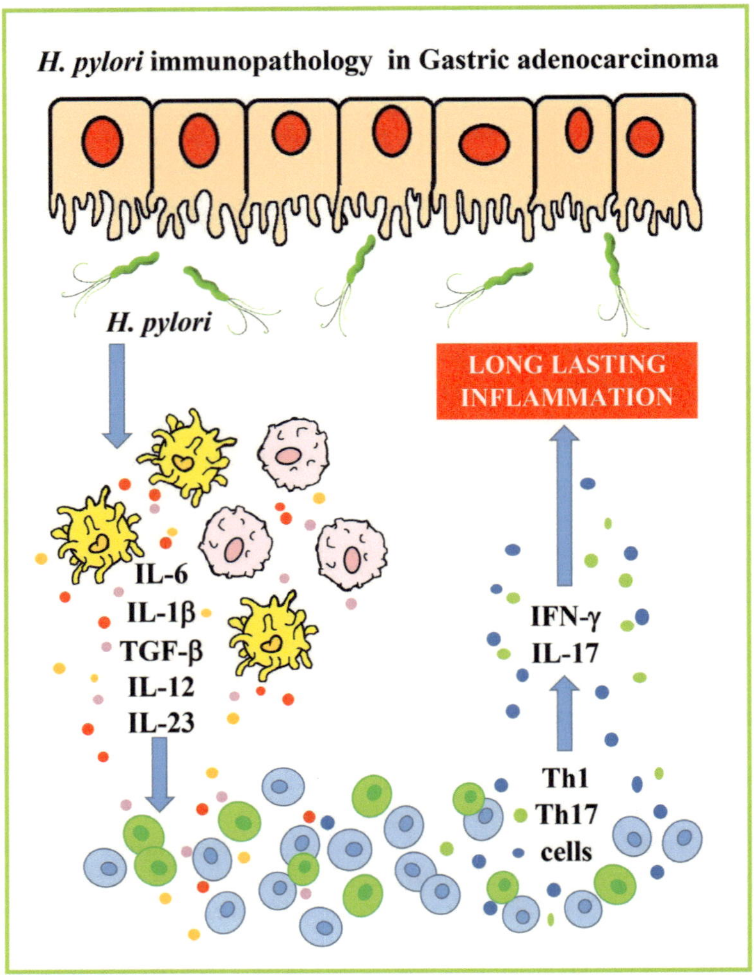

Figure 4.
Th17 and Th1 immunopathology in gastric adenocarcinoma.

Th17 immune response is directly driven by several *H. pylori* antigens such as the above-mentioned HP0175, HP1454, CagY. T cells specific for HP0175, HP1454, CagY, and other *H. pylori* antigens, are activated in the stomach by *H. pylori* and secrete IL-17. The number of *H. pylori*-specific Th17 cells present in the gastric mucosa is significantly elevated in patients with gastric premalignant and malignant lesions than in patients with uncomplicated chronic gastritis. Thus *H. pylori* drives abnormal and long-lasting IL-17 production in some predisposed individuals leading to gastric cancer [33, 36, 102, 110]. All these results point out that *H. pylori* is strongly able to promote Th17 and Th1 inflammation in gastric cancer (**Figure 4**).

6. Conclusions

H. pylori infection is the primary reason for gastroduodenal issues, however, only a small portion of *H. pylori*-positive individuals will experience long-term and serious conditions like gastric cancer, B cell lymphoma, autoimmune gastritis, or peptic ulcer. The type of host immune response against the bacterium is crucial for the outcome of the infection. We investigated gastric immune responses in patients with gastric cancer, gastric autoimmunity, peptic ulcer, and gastric lymphoma. A predominant immune-pathological Th1 response, characterized by high IFN-γ, TNF-α, and IL-12 production is a hallmark of *H. pylori* infection, whereas combined secretion of both Th1 and Th2 cytokines are present in *H. pylori* infection with uncomplicated gastritis. We showed that a polarized gastric Th1/Th17 response is built-up in *H. pylori*-positive subjects with gastric adenocarcinoma, as well as in patients with gastric intestinal metaplasia and dysplasia (IM, DYS). In *H. pylori*-infected patients, autoimmune gastritis occurs due to cytolytic T cells that are activated following the cross-recognition of different epitopes of *H. pylori* proteins and H^+/K^+-ATPase autoantigen via molecular mimicry. In *H. pylori*-related low-grade gastric mucosa-associated lymphoid tissue (MALT) lymphoma, the neoplastic B cells proliferate in response to *H. pylori* only in the presence of autologous T cells that are essential for B cell proliferation. Different *H. pylori* antigens, such as Cag Y drive gastric inflammation in low-grade MALT lymphoma. Gastric T cells infiltrating MALT lymphoma mucosa have impaired ability to kill B cells through perforin and Fas-FasL pathways, leading to excessive support for B cell growth. This indicates that uncontrolled *H. pylori*-induced activation of T lymphocytes can contribute to the development and progression of low-grade B cell lymphoma. The International Agency for Research on Cancer has categorized *H. pylori* as a type I oncogenic factor for gastric adenocarcinoma.

The development of stomach cancer is a multi-step process that can take many years and can progress to pre-cancerous stages like gastric intestinal metaplasia and dysplasia (IM and DYS) before becoming a tumor. We recently analyzed the serum IL-17A levels in individuals with gastric IM and DYS, and observed a significant rise in IL-17A serum levels among these patients. Based on the results obtained so far, we propose that testing serum IL-17A levels could help in handling *H. pylori*-infected subjects and possibly even in predicting the onset of gastric cancer.

Acknowledgements

We thank the Italian Ministry of University and Research (PRIN project - Grant n. 2010P3S8BR_005) for supporting our studies. We thank Mary Wilkins for the English editing of the manuscript.

Conflict of interest

The authors certify that there is not any actual or potential conflict of interest.

Author details

Mario M. D'Elios* and Chiara Della Bella
Department of Molecular and Developmental Medicine, University of Siena, Siena, Italy

*Address all correspondence to: delios@unisi.it

References

[1] Marshall BJ, Warren JR. Unidentified curved bacilli in the stomach of patients with gastritis and peptic ulceration. Lancet. 1984;**1**(8390):1311-1315. DOI: 10.1016/s0140-6736(84)91816-6

[2] Robinson K, Atherton JC. The spectrum of helicobacter-mediated diseases. Annual Review of Pathology. 2021;**16**:123-144. DOI: 10.1146/annurev-pathol-032520-024949

[3] Parsonnet J, Friedman GD, Vandersteen DP, Chang Y, Vogelman JH, Orentreich N, et al. *Helicobacter pylori* infection and the risk of gastric carcinoma. The New England Journal of Medicine. 1991;**325**(16):1127-1131. DOI: 10.1056/NEJM199110173251603

[4] Nomura A, Stemmermann GN, Chyou PH, Kato I, Perez-Perez GI, Blaser MJ. *Helicobacter pylori* infection and gastric carcinoma among Japanese Americans in Hawaii. The New England Journal of Medicine. 1991;**325**(16):1132-1136. DOI: 10.1056/NEJM199110173251604

[5] Amieva M, Peek RM Jr. Pathobiology of *Helicobacter pylori*-induced gastric cancer. Gastroenterology. 2016;**150**(1):64-78. DOI: 10.1053/j.gastro.2015.09.004

[6] Canzian F, Rizzato C, Stein A, Flores-Luna L, Camorlinga-Ponce M, Mendez-Tenorio A, et al. Phylogenetic origin of *Helicobacter pylori* pathogenicity island and risk of stomach cancer and high-grade premalignant gastric lesions. European Journal of Cancer Prevention. 2023;**32**(3):301-304. DOI: 10.1097/CEJ.0000000000000779

[7] Wotherspoon AC, Doglioni C, Diss TC, Pan L, Moschini A, de Boni M, et al. Regression of primary low-grade B-cell gastric lymphoma of mucosa-associated lymphoid tissue type after eradication of *Helicobacter pylori*. Lancet. 1993;**342**(8871):575-577. DOI: 10.1016/0140-6736(93)91409-f

[8] Floch P, Mégraud F, Lehours P. *Helicobacter pylori* strains and gastric MALT lymphoma. Toxins (Basel). 2017;**9**(4):132. DOI: 10.3390/toxins9040132

[9] Rossi D, Bertoni F, Zucca E. Marginal-zone lymphomas. The New England Journal of Medicine. 2022;**385**(6):568-581. DOI: 10.1056/NEJMra2102568

[10] D'Elios MM, Appelmelk BJ, Amedei A, Bergman MP, Del Prete G. Gastric autoimmunity: The role of *Helicobacter pylori* and molecular mimicry. Trends in Molecular Medicine. 2004;**10**(7):316-323. DOI: 10.1016/j.molmed.2004.06.001

[11] Fox JG, Wang TC. Inflammation, atrophy, and gastric cancer. The Journal of Clinical Investigation. 2007;**117**(1):60-69. DOI: 10.1172/JCI30111

[12] Schistosomes, liver flukes and *Helicobacter pylori*. IARC Monographs on the Evaluation of Carcinogenic Risks to Humans. 1994;**61**:1-241

[13] Choi IJ, Kim CG, Lee JY, Kim YI, Kook MC, Park B, et al. Family history of gastric cancer and *Helicobacter pylori* treatment. The New England Journal of Medicine. 2020;**382**(5):427-436. DOI: 10.1056/NEJMoa1909666

[14] Kuipers EJ, Sipponen P. *Helicobacter pylori* eradication for the prevention of gastric cancer. Helicobacter. 2006;**11**(Suppl 1):52-57. DOI: 10.1111/j.1478-405X.2006.00425.x

[15] Lee YC, Dore MP, Graham DY. Diagnosis and treatment of *Helicobacter pylori* infection. Annual Review of Medicine. 2022;**73**:183-195. DOI: 10.1146/annurev-med-042220-020814

[16] Choi IJ, Kook MC, Kim YI, Cho SJ, Lee JY, Kim CG, et al. *Helicobacter pylori* therapy for the prevention of metachronous gastric cancer. The New England Journal of Medicine. 2018;**378**(12):1085-1095. DOI: 10.1056/NEJMoa1708423

[17] Kalali B, Mejías-Luque R, Javaheri A, Gerhard MH. *Pylori* virulence factors: Influence on immune system and pathology. Mediators of Inflammation. 2014;**2014**:426309. DOI: 10.1155/2014/426309

[18] Moss SF, Blaser MJ. Mechanisms of disease: Inflammation and the origins of cancer. Nature Clinical Practice. Oncology. 2005;**2**(2):90-97; quiz 1 p following 113. DOI: 10.1038/ncponc0081

[19] Molinari M, Salio M, Galli C, Norais N, Rappuoli R, Lanzavecchia A, et al. Selective inhibition of Ii-dependent antigen presentation by *Helicobacter pylori* toxin VacA. The Journal of Experimental Medicine. 1998;**187**(1):135-140. DOI: 10.1084/jem.187.1.135

[20] Gebert B, Fischer W, Weiss E, Hoffmann R, Haas R. *Helicobacter pylori* vacuolating cytotoxin inhibits T lymphocyte activation. Science. 2003;**301**(5636):1099-1102. DOI: 10.1126/science.1086871

[21] Boncristiano M, Paccani SR, Barone S, Ulivieri C, Patrussi L, Ilver D, et al. The *Helicobacter pylori* vacuolating toxin inhibits T cell activation by two independent mechanisms. The Journal of Experimental Medicine. 2003;**198**(12):1887-1897. DOI: 10.1084/jem.20030621

[22] Schmees C, Prinz C, Treptau T, Rad R, Hengst L, Voland P, et al. Inhibition of T-cell proliferation by *Helicobacter pylori* gamma-glutamyl transpeptidase. Gastroenterology. 2007;**132**(5):1820-1833. DOI: 10.1053/j.gastro.2007.02.031

[23] Amedei A, Munari F, Della Bella C, Niccolai E, Benagiano M, Bencini L, et al. *Helicobacter pylori* HP0175 promotes the production of IL-23, IL-6, IL-1b and TGF-b. European Journal of Inflammation. 2013;**11**(1):261-268. DOI: 10.1177/1721727X1301100127

[24] Amedei A, Cappon A, Codolo G, Cabrelle A, Polenghi A, Benagiano M, et al. The neutrophil-activating protein of *Helicobacter pylori* promotes Th1 immune responses. The Journal of Clinical Investigation. 2006;**116**(4):1092-1101. DOI: 10.1172/JCI27177. Epub 2006 Mar 16

[25] Crabtree JE, Peichl P, Wyatt JI, Stachl U, Lindley IJ. Gastric interleukin-8 and IgA IL-8 autoantibodies in *Helicobacter pylori* infection. Scandinavian Journal of Immunology. 1993;**37**(1):65-70. DOI: 10.1111/j.1365-3083.1993.tb01666.x

[26] Kaparakis M, Philpott DJ, Ferrero RL. Mammalian NLR proteins; discriminating foe from friend. Immunology and Cell Biology. 2007;**85**(6):495-502. DOI: 10.1038/sj.icb.7100105. Epub 2007 Aug 7

[27] D'Elios MM, Manghetti M, Almerigogna F, Amedei A, Costa F, Burroni D, et al. Different cytokine profile and antigen-specificity repertoire in *Helicobacter pylori*-specific T cell clones from the antrum of chronic gastritis patients with or without peptic ulcer. European Journal of Immunology. 1997;**27**(7):1751-1755. DOI: 10.1002/eji.1830270723

[28] Meyer F, Wilson KT, James SP. Modulation of innate cytokine responses by products of *Helicobacter pylori*. Infection and Immunity. 2000;**68**(11):6265-6272. DOI: 10.1128/IAI.68.11.6265-6272.2000

[29] Della, Bella C, D'Elios S, Coletta S, Benagiano M, Azzurri A, Cianchi F, et al. Increased IL-17A serum levels and gastric Th17 cells in *Helicobacter pylori*-infected patients with gastric premalignant lesions. Cancers (Basel). 2023;**15**(6):1662. DOI: 10.3390/cancers15061662

[30] Vinagre RMDF, Vinagre IDF, Vilar-E-Silva A, Fecury AA, Martins LC. *Helicobacter pylori* infection and immune profile of patients with different gastroduodenal diseases. Arquivos de Gastroenterologia. 2018;**55**(2):122-127. DOI: 10.1590/S0004-2803.201800000-21

[31] Weaver CT, Hatton RD, Mangan PR, Harrington LE. IL-17 family cytokines and the expanding diversity of effector T cell lineages. Annual Review of Immunology. 2007;**25**:821-852. DOI: 10.1146/annurev.immunol.25.022106.141557

[32] Korn T, Bettelli E, Oukka M, Kuchroo VK. IL-17 and Th17 cells. Annual Review of Immunology. 2009;**27**:485-517. DOI: 10.1146/annurev.immunol.021908.132710

[33] Capitani N, Codolo G, Vallese F, Minervini G, Grassi A, Cianchi F, et al. The lipoprotein HP1454 of *Helicobacter pylori* regulates T-cell response by shaping T-cell receptor signalling. Cellular Microbiology. 2019;**21**(5):e13006. DOI: 10.1111/cmi.13006

[34] Shi Y, Liu XF, Zhuang Y, Zhang JY, Liu T, Yin Z, et al. *Helicobacter pylori*-induced Th17 responses modulate Th1 cell responses, benefit bacterial growth, and contribute to pathology in mice. Journal of Immunology. 2010;**184**(9):5121-5129. DOI: 10.4049/jimmunol.0901115

[35] Kang JH, Park S, Rho J, Hong EJ, Cho YE, Won YS, et al. IL-17A promotes *Helicobacter pylori*-induced gastric carcinogenesis via interactions with IL-17RC. Gastric Cancer. 2023;**26**(1):82-94. DOI: 10.1007/s10120-022-01342-5. Epub 2022 Sep 20

[36] Della Bella C, Soluri MF, Puccio S, Benagiano M, Grassi A, Bitetti J, et al. The *Helicobacter pylori* CagY protein drives gastric Th1 and Th17 inflammation and B cell proliferation in gastric MALT lymphoma. International Journal of Molecular Sciences. 2021;**22**(17):9459. DOI: 10.3390/ijms22179459

[37] D'Elios MM, Manghetti M, De Carli M, Costa F, Baldari CT, Burroni D, et al. T helper 1 effector cells specific for *Helicobacter pylori* in the gastric antrum of patients with peptic ulcer disease. Journal of Immunology. 1997;**158**(2):962-967

[38] Sommer F, Faller G, Konturek P, Kirchner T, Hahn EG, Zeus J, et al. Antrum- and corpus mucosa-infiltrating CD4(+) lymphocytes in *Helicobacter pylori* gastritis display a Th1 phenotype. Infection and Immunity. 1998;**66**(11):5543-5546. DOI: 10.1128/IAI.66.11.5543-5546.1998

[39] Bamford KB, Fan X, Crowe SE, Leary JF, Gourley WK, Luthra GK, et al. Lymphocytes in the human gastric mucosa during *Helicobacter pylori* have a T helper cell 1 phenotype. Gastroenterology. 1998;**114**(3):482-492. DOI: 10.1016/s0016-5085(98)70531-1

[40] de Jonge R, Kuipers EJ, Langeveld SC, Loffeld RJ, Stoof J,

van Vliet AH, et al. The *Helicobacter pylori* plasticity region locus jhp0947-jhp0949 is associated with duodenal ulcer disease and interleukin-12 production in monocyte cells. FEMS Immunology and Medical Microbiology. 2004;**41**(2):161-167. DOI: 10.1016/j.femsim.2004.03.003

[41] Lehmann FS, Terracciano L, Carena I, Baeriswyl C, Drewe J, Tornillo L, et al. *In situ* correlation of cytokine secretion and apoptosis in *Helicobacter pylori*-associated gastritis. American Journal of Physiology. Gastrointestinal and Liver Physiology. 2002;**283**(2):G481-G488. DOI: 10.1152/ajpgi.00422.2001

[42] Wen S, Felley CP, Bouzourene H, Reimers M, Michetti P, Pan-Hammarström Q. Inflammatory gene profiles in gastric mucosa during *Helicobacter pylori* infection in humans. Journal of Immunology. 2004;**172**(4):2595-2606. DOI: 10.4049/jimmunol.172.4.2595

[43] Pellicanò A, Sebkova L, Monteleone G, Guarnieri G, Imeneo M, Pallone F, et al. Interleukin-12 drives the Th1 signaling pathway in *Helicobacter pylori*-infected human gastric mucosa. Infection and Immunity. 2007;**75**(4):1738-1744. DOI: 10.1128/IAI.01446-06

[44] Touati E, Michel V, Thiberge JM, Wuscher N, Huerre M, Labigne A. Chronic *Helicobacter pylori* infections induce gastric mutations in mice. Gastroenterology. 2003;**124**(5):1408-1419. DOI: 10.1016/s0016-5085(03)00266-x

[45] McCune A, Lane A, Murray L, Harvey I, Nair P, Donovan J, et al. Reduced risk of atopic disorders in adults with *Helicobacter pylori* infection. European Journal of Gastroenterology & Hepatology. 2003;**15**(6):637-640. DOI:10.1097/00042737-200306000-00010

[46] Codolo G, Coletta S, D'Elios MM, de Bernard M. HP-NAP of *Helicobacter pylori*: The power of the immunomodulation. Frontiers in Immunology. 2022;**13**:944139. DOI: 10.3389/fimmu.2022.944139

[47] Borbet TC, Zhang X, Müller A, Blaser MJ. The role of the changing human microbiome in the asthma pandemic. The Journal of Allergy and Clinical Immunology. 2019;**144**(6):1457-1466. DOI: 10.1016/j.jaci.2019.10.022

[48] Chen Y, Blaser MJ. Inverse associations of *Helicobacter pylori* with asthma and allergy. Archives of Internal Medicine. 2007;**167**(8):821-827. DOI: 10.1001/archinte.167.8.821

[49] Jaka H, Smith SI. Forty years of *H. pylori*: The African perspective. Digestive Diseases. 2023;**42**(2):161-165. DOI: 10.1159/000535263

[50] Holcombe C. *Helicobacter pylori*: The African enigma. Gut. 1992;**33**(4):429-431. DOI: 10.1136/gut.33.4.429

[51] D'Elios MM, Andersen LP, Del Prete G. Inflammation and host reponse. Current Opinion in Gastroenterology Online. 1998;**14**(suppl 1):S15-S19

[52] Mejías-Luque R, Gerhard M. Immune evasion strategies and persistence of *Helicobacter pylori*. Current Topics in Microbiology and Immunology. 2017;**400**:53-71. DOI: 10.1007/978-3-319-50520-6_3

[53] Cadamuro AC, Rossi AF, Maniezzo NM, Silva AE. *Helicobacter pylori* infection: Host immune response, implications on gene expression and microRNAs. World Journal of Gastroenterology. 2014;**20**(6):1424-1437. DOI: 10.3748/wjg.v20.i6.1424

[54] Merrell DS, Falkow S. Frontal and stealth attack strategies in microbial pathogenesis. Nature. 2004;**430**(6996):250-256. DOI: 10.1038/nature02760

[55] Correa P, Haenszel W, Cuello C, Tannenbaum S, Archer M. A model for gastric cancer epidemiology. Lancet. 1975;**2**(7924):58-60. DOI: 10.1016/s0140-6736(75)90498-5

[56] Correa P. Human gastric carcinogenesis: A multistep and multifactorial process—first American Cancer Society award lecture on cancer epidemiology and prevention. Cancer Research. 1992;**52**(24):6735-6740

[57] Huang KK, Ramnarayanan K, Zhu F, Srivastava S, Xu C, Tan ALK, et al. Genomic and epigenomic profiling of high-risk intestinal metaplasia reveals molecular determinants of progression to gastric cancer. Cancer Cell. 2018;**33**(1):137-150.e5. DOI: 10.1016/j.ccell.2017.11.018

[58] Costa L, Corre S, Michel V, Le Luel K, Fernandes J, Ziveri J, et al. USF1 defect drives p53 degradation during *Helicobacter pylori* infection and accelerates gastric carcinogenesis. Gut. 2020;**69**(9):1582-1591. DOI: 10.1136/gutjnl-2019-318640

[59] Guo Y, Huang A, Hu C, Zhou Y, Zhang X, Czajkowsky DM, et al. Complex clonal mosaicism within microdissected intestinal metaplastic glands without concurrent gastric cancer. Journal of Medical Genetics. 2016;**53**(9):643-646. DOI: 10.1136/jmedgenet-2016-103872

[60] Dixon BREA, Hossain R, Patel RV, Algood HMS. Th17 cells in *Helicobacter pylori* infection: A dichotomy of help and harm. Infection and Immunity. 2019;**87**(11):e00363-e00319. DOI: 10.1128/IAI.00363-19

[61] Toh BH, van Driel IR, Gleeson PA. Pernicious anemia. The New England Journal of Medicine. 1997;**337**(20):1441-1448. DOI: 10.1056/NEJM199711133372007

[62] Bergman MP, Vandenbroucke-Grauls CM, Appelmelk BJ, D'Elios MM, Amedei A, Azzurri A, et al. The story so far: *Helicobacter pylori* and gastric autoimmunity. International Reviews of Immunology. 2005;**24**(1-2):63-91. DOI: 10.1080/08830180590884648

[63] Stolte M, Baumann K, Bethke B, Ritter M, Lauer E, Eidt H. Active autoimmune gastritis without total atrophy of the glands. Zeitschrift für Gastroenterologie. 1992;**30**(10):729-735

[64] Stolte M, Meier E, Meining A. Cure of autoimmune gastritis by *Helicobacter pylori* eradication in a 21-year-old male. Zeitschrift für Gastroenterologie. 1998;**36**(8):641-643

[65] Tucci A, Poli L, Tosetti C, Biasco G, Grigioni W, Varoli O, et al. Reversal of fundic atrophy after eradication of *Helicobacter pylori*. The American Journal of Gastroenterology. 1998;**93**(9):1425-1431. DOI: 10.1111/j.1572-0241.1998.00454.x

[66] Faller G, Steininger H, Eck M, Hensen J, Hann EG, Kirchner T. Antigastric autoantibodies in *Helicobacter pylori* gastritis: Prevalence, in-situ binding sites and clues for clinical relevance. Virchows Archiv. 1996;**427**(5):483-486. DOI: 10.1007/BF00199508

[67] Faller G, Steininger H, Kränzlein J, Maul H, Kerkau T, Hensen J, et al. Antigastric autoantibodies in *Helicobacter pylori* infection: Implications of histological and clinical parameters of gastritis. Gut. 1997;**41**(5):619-623. DOI: 10.1136/gut.41.5.619

[68] Negrini R, Lisato L, Zanella I, Cavazzini L, Gullini S, Villanacci V, et al. *Helicobacter pylori* infection induces antibodies cross-reacting with human gastric mucosa. Gastroenterology. 1991;**101**(2):437-445. DOI: 10.1016/0016-5085(91)90023-e

[69] Negrini R, Savio A, Poiesi C, Appelmelk BJ, Buffoli F, Paterlini A, et al. Antigenic mimicry between *Helicobacter pylori* and gastric mucosa in the pathogenesis of body atrophic gastritis. Gastroenterology. 1996;**111**(3):655-665. DOI: 10.1053/gast.1996.v111.pm8780570

[70] Steininger H, Faller G, Dewald E, Brabletz T, Jung A, Kirchner T. Apoptosis in chronic gastritis and its correlation with antigastric autoantibodies. Virchows Archiv. 1998;**433**(1):13-18. DOI: 10.1007/s004280050210

[71] Toh BH, Sentry JW, Alderuccio F. The causative H+/K+ ATPase antigen in the pathogenesis of autoimmune gastritis. Immunology Today. 2000;**21**(7):348-354. DOI: 10.1016/s0167-5699(00)01653-4

[72] Claeys D, Faller G, Appelmelk BJ, Negrini R, Kirchner T. The gastric H^+, K^+-ATPase is a major autoantigen in chronic *Helicobacter pylori* gastritis with body mucosa atrophy. Gastroenterology. 1998;**115**(2):340-347. DOI: 10.1016/s0016-5085(98)70200-8

[73] Appelmelk BJ, Faller G, Claeys D, Kirchner T, Vandenbroucke-Grauls CM. Bugs on trial: The case of *Helicobacter pylori* and autoimmunity. Immunology Today. 1998;**19**(7):296-299. DOI: 10.1016/s0167-5699(98)01281-x

[74] Amedei A, Bergman MP, Appelmelk BJ, Azzurri A, Benagiano M, Tamburini C, et al. Molecular mimicry between *Helicobacter pylori* antigens and H^+, K^+-adenosine triphosphatase in human gastric autoimmunity. The Journal of Experimental Medicine. 2003;**198**(8):1147-1156. DOI: 10.1084/jem.20030530

[75] D'Elios MM, Bergman MP, Azzurri A, Amedei A, Benagiano M, De Pont JJ, et al. H^+, K^+-ATPase (proton pump) is the target autoantigen of Th1-type cytotoxic T cells in autoimmune gastritis. Gastroenterology. 2001;**120**(2):377-386. DOI: 10.1053/gast.2001.21187

[76] Bergman MP, Amedei A, D'Elios MM, Azzurri A, Benagiano M, Tamburini C, et al. Characterization of H^+, K^+-ATPase T cell epitopes in human autoimmune gastritis. European Journal of Immunology. 2003;**33**(2):539-545. DOI: 10.1002/immu.200310030. Erratum in: Eur J Immunol. 2003 Apr; 33(4):1139

[77] Houghton J, Macera-Bloch LS, Harrison L, Kim KH, Korah RM. Tumor necrosis factor alpha and interleukin 1beta up-regulate gastric mucosal Fas antigen expression in *Helicobacter pylori* infection. Infection and Immunity. 2000;**68**(3):1189-1195. DOI: 10.1128/IAI.68.3.1189-1195.2000

[78] Wang J, Fan X, Lindholm C, Bennett M, O'Connoll J, Shanahan F, et al. *Helicobacter pylori* modulates lymphoepithelial cell interactions leading to epithelial cell damage through Fas/Fas ligand interactions. Infection and Immunity. 2000;**68**(7):4303-4311. DOI: 10.1128/IAI.68.7.4303-4311.2000

[79] A clinical evaluation of the International Lymphoma Study Group classification of non-Hodgkin's lymphoma. The non-Hodgkin's lymphoma classification project. Blood. 1997;**89**(11):3909-3918

[80] Du MQ. MALT lymphoma: Recent advances in aetiology and molecular

genetics. Journal of Clinical and Experimental Hematopathology. 2007;**47**(2):31-42. DOI: 10.3960/jslrt.47.31

[81] Isaacson P, Wright DH. Malignant lymphoma of mucosa-associated lymphoid tissue. A distinctive type of B-cell lymphoma. Cancer. 1983;**52**(8):1410-1416. DOI: 10.1002/1097-0142(19831015)52:8<1410::aid-cncr2820520813>3.0.co;2-3

[82] Wotherspoon AC, Ortiz-Hidalgo C, Falzon MR, Isaacson PG. *Helicobacter pylori*-associated gastritis and primary B-cell gastric lymphoma. Lancet. 1991;**338**(8776):1175-1176. DOI: 10.1016/0140-6736(91)92035-z

[83] Hussell T, Isaacson PG, Crabtree JE, Spencer J. The response of cells from low-grade B-cell gastric lymphomas of mucosa-associated lymphoid tissue to *Helicobacter pylori*. Lancet. 1993;**342**(8871):571-574. DOI: 10.1016/0140-6736(93)91408-e

[84] Hussell T, Isaacson PG, Crabtree JE, Spencer J. *Helicobacter pylori*-specific tumour-infiltrating T cells provide contact dependent help for the growth of malignant B cells in low-grade gastric lymphoma of mucosa-associated lymphoid tissue. The Journal of Pathology. 1996;**178**(2):122-127. DOI: 10.1002/(SICI)1096-9896(199602)178:2<122::AID-PATH486>3.0.CO;2-D

[85] Greiner A, Knörr C, Qin Y, Sebald W, Schimpl A, Banchereau J, et al. Low-grade B cell lymphomas of mucosa-associated lymphoid tissue (MALT-type) require CD40-mediated signaling and Th2-type cytokines for *in vitro* growth and differentiation. The American Journal of Pathology. 1997;**150**(5):1583-1593

[86] D'Elios MM, Amedei A, Manghetti M, Costa F, Baldari CT, Quazi AS, et al. Impaired T-cell regulation of B-cell growth in *Helicobacter pylori*—related gastric low-grade MALT lymphoma. Gastroenterology. 1999;**117**(5):1105-1112. DOI: 10.1016/s0016-5085(99)70395-1. 2002; 2(10): 735-47. DOI: 10.1038/nri911

[87] Smyth MJ, Thia KY, Street SE, MacGregor D, Godfrey DI, Trapani JA. Perforin-mediated cytotoxicity is critical for surveillance of spontaneous lymphoma. The Journal of Experimental Medicine. 2000;**192**(5):755-760. DOI: 10.1084/jem.192.5.755

[88] Street SE, Trapani JA, MacGregor D, Smyth MJ. Suppression of lymphoma and epithelial malignancies effected by interferon gamma. The Journal of Experimental Medicine. 2002;**196**(1):129-134. DOI: 10.1084/jem.20020063

[89] Street SE, Hayakawa Y, Zhan Y, Lew AM, MacGregor D, Jamieson AM, et al. Innate immune surveillance of spontaneous B cell lymphomas by natural killer cells and gammadelta T cells. The Journal of Experimental Medicine. 2004;**199**(6):879-884. DOI: 10.1084/jem.20031981

[90] Clementi R, Locatelli F, Dupré L, Garaventa A, Emmi L, Bregni M, et al. A proportion of patients with lymphoma may harbor mutations of the perforin gene. Blood. 2005;**105**(11):4424-4428. DOI: 10.1182/blood-2004-04-1477

[91] Lehours P, Zheng Z, Skoglund A, Mégraud F, Engstrand L. Is there a link between the lipopolysaccharide of *Helicobacter pylori* gastric MALT lymphoma associated strains and lymphoma pathogenesis? PLoS One. 2009;**4**(10):e7297. DOI: 10.1371/journal.pone.0007297

[92] Lehours P, Dupouy S, Bergey B, Ruskoné-Foumestraux A, Delchier JC, Rad R, et al. Identification of a genetic marker of *Helicobacter pylori* strains involved in gastric extranodal marginal zone B cell lymphoma of the MALT-type. Gut. 2004;**53**(7):931-937. DOI: 10.1136/gut.2003.028811

[93] Correa P, Piazuelo MB. The gastric precancerous cascade. Journal of Digestive Diseases. 2012;**13**(1):2-9. DOI: 10.1111/j.1751-2980.2011.00550.x

[94] van Loo G, Bertrand MJM. Death by TNF: A road to inflammation. Nature Reviews. Immunology. 2023;**23**(5):289-303. DOI: 10.1038/s41577-022-00792-3

[95] Ohno M, Kato M, Nakamura T, Saitoh Y. Gene expression for tumor necrosis factor alpha and its production in gastric cancer patients. Japanese Journal of Cancer Research. 1994;**85**(10):1029-1034. DOI: 10.1111/j.1349-7006.1994.tb02901.x

[96] El-Omar EM, Carrington M, Chow WH, McColl KE, Bream JH, Young HA, et al. Interleukin-1 polymorphisms associated with increased risk of gastric cancer. Nature. 2000;**404**(6776):398-402. DOI: 10.1038/35006081. Erratum in: Nature 2001; 412(6842):99

[97] Salama NR, Hartung ML, Müller A. Life in the human stomach: Persistence strategies of the bacterial pathogen *Helicobacter pylori*. Nature Reviews. Microbiology. 2013;**11**(6):385-399. DOI: 10.1038/nrmicro3016

[98] Wroblewski LE, Peek RM Jr, Wilson KT. *Helicobacter pylori* and gastric cancer: Factors that modulate disease risk. Clinical Microbiology Reviews. 2010;**23**(4):713-739. DOI: 10.1128/CMR.00011-10

[99] Moyat M, Velin D. Immune responses to *Helicobacter pylori* infection. World Journal of Gastroenterology. 2014;**20**(19):5583-5593. DOI: 10.3748/wjg.v20.i19.5583

[100] Greten FR, Grivennikov SI. Inflammation and cancer: Triggers, mechanisms, and consequences. Immunity. 2019;**51**(1):27-41. DOI: 10.1016/j.immuni.2019.06.025

[101] Zhang B, Rong G, Wei H, Zhang M, Bi J, Ma L, et al. The prevalence of Th17 cells in patients with gastric cancer. Biochemical and Biophysical Research Communications. 2008;**374**(3):533-537. DOI: 10.1016/j.bbrc.2008.07.060

[102] El-Omar EM, Carrington M, Chow WH, McColl KE, Bream JH, Young HA, et al. The role of interleukin-1 polymorphisms in the pathogenesis of gastric cancer. Nature. 2001;**412**(6842):99. DOI: 10.1038/35083631

[103] Luzza F, Parrello T, Monteleone G, Sebkova L, Romano M, Zarrilli R, et al. Up-regulation of IL-17 is associated with bioactive IL-8 expression in *Helicobacter pylori*-infected human gastric mucosa. Journal of Immunology. 2000;**165**(9):5332-5337. DOI: 10.4049/jimmunol.165.9.5332

[104] Della Bella C, Antico A, Panozzo MP, Capitani N, Petrone L, Benagiano M, et al. Gastric Th17 cells specific for H+/K+-ATPase and serum IL-17 signature in gastric autoimmunity. Frontiers in Immunology. 2022;**13**:952674. DOI: 10.3389/fimmu.2022.952674

[105] International Agency for the Research on Cancer (WHO). Global Cancer Observatory – Globocan [Internet]. Lyon, France: International Agency for the Research on Cancer

(WHO); 2024. Available from: https://gco.iarc.fr/ [Accessed: January 1, 2024]

[106] Alikhani M, Esmaeili M, Tashakoripour M, Mohagheghi MA, Eshagh Hosseini M, Touati E, et al. Alteration in serum levels of tumor necrosis factor alpha is associated with histopathologic progression of gastric cancer. Iranian Biomedical Journal. 2023;**27**(1):72-78. DOI: 10.52547/ibj.3847

[107] Amedei A, Niccolai E, Della Bella C, Cianchi F, Trallori G, Benagiano M, et al. Characterization of tumor antigen peptide-specific T cells isolated from the neoplastic tissue of patients with gastric adenocarcinoma. Cancer Immunology, Immunotherapy. 2009;**58**(11):1819-1830. DOI: 10.1007/s00262-009-0693-8

[108] Fragoulis GE, Siebert S, McInnes IB. Therapeutic targeting of IL-17 and IL-23 cytokines in immune-mediated diseases. Annual Review of Medicine. 2016;**67**:337-353. DOI: 10.1146/annurev-med-051914-021944. Epub 2015 Nov 4

[109] Sun K, Xu R, Ma F, Yang N, Li Y, Sun X, et al. scRNA-seq of gastric tumor shows complex intercellular interaction with an alternative T cell exhaustion trajectory. Nature Communications. 2022;**13**(1):4943. DOI: 10.1038/s41467-022-32627-z

[110] Li S, Cong X, Gao H, Lan X, Li Z, Wang W, et al. Tumor-associated neutrophils induce EMT by IL-17a to promote migration and invasion in gastric cancer cells. Journal of Experimental & Clinical Cancer Research. 2019;**38**(1):6. DOI: 10.1186/s13046-018-1003-0

Chapter 3

Invasive and Non-Invasive Methods of Diagnosing *H. pylori* Infection: A Review of Current Practice

Taylor Fontenot and Annabel E. Barber

Abstract

H. pylori infection can be diagnosed using both noninvasive and invasive methods. There is no one gold standard test that is used for diagnosis. Invasive methods of diagnosis involve endoscopy with biopsy, histologic examination, culture, and rapid urease testing. There are certain clinical situations that are appropriate for noninvasive testing and invasive testing. Choosing the appropriate method of diagnosis is dependent upon multiple factors including pretest probability of Infection as well as cost-effectiveness and availability. The aim of this chapter is to discuss the current options of diagnosis, when invasive testing is indicated, and the interpretation of the results obtained.

Keywords: *H. pylori*, endoscopy, invasive testing, peptic ulcer disease, urease, culture, histology

1. Introduction

H. pylori infection remains the most common chronic bacterial infection in humans. It is estimated that half of the world's population is infected with *H. pylori*, making its clinical and global impact of great significance. It is the leading cause of gastritis and peptic ulcer disease. Additionally, prolonged colonization and infection can progress to development of gastric carcinoma. *H. pylori* infection is also associated with gastric lymphoma. Protective factors against *H. pylori* infection include adequate nutritional status, especially enteral consumption of fruits, vegetables, and foods with high vitamin C content. Higher prevalence of *H. pylori* infection has been linked to poor sanitation practices, low socioeconomic class, and crowded or high-density living conditions, facilitating intrafamilial and institutional transmission [1]. In general, the most plausible mode of transmission is via oral-oral (i.e., emesis or saliva) or fecal-oral route. Oral-oral transmission between persons is supported by higher incidence of infection among institutionalized individuals and clustering of familial *H. pylori* infections [1]. Fecal contamination of water supply in developing regions is a significant source of infection as well. The above modes of transmission form the basis of detection of *H. pylori* through the various non-invasive methods of diagnosis. Treatment of *H. pylori*-related illness, especially ulcers and gastric cancers, contributes significantly to the financial burden of healthcare globally. In some regions with high prevalence rates, screening programs have been developed to target at-risk populations to detect and treat *H. pylori* infections early, aiming to prevent sequelae of disease. The aim of this chapter will be to discuss the salient points regarding the history of *H. pylori* and its clinical relevance, indications for testing, methods of diagnosis, and confirmation of bacterial eradication.

2. Historical background of *H. pylori*

The discovery of *Helicobacter pylori* stands as a testament to the transformative power of scientific investigation and serves as a model for challenging established beliefs in medicine. Prior to discovery, the pathology of peptic ulcer disease was thought to be a result of excess acid production secondary to endogenous stress from catecholamine induced acid production and exogenous exposure of gastric mucosa to food with high acid content. Drs Marshall and Warren were credited with discovering the link between *H. pylori* infection and peptic ulcers and gastric cancer in 1984 [2]. They suspected that a bacterium was the underlying cause, given observations of a spiral-spaced bacteria present in gastric biopsy samples from patients suffering from gastritis and peptic ulcers. Many prior studies attempting to prove the link in animal models were unsuccessful in establishing the association between *H. pylori* colonization and pathologic disease. In their Nobel Prize-winning landmark paper, Marshall conducted the famous self-experiment in which he administered a solution containing a suspension of cultured *H. pylori* organisms. He documented onset of symptoms within 5 days of ingestion and further confirmed progression of pathology with endoscopic evaluation. Their work revolutionized modern medicine, leading to a paradigm shift in gastroenterology.

2.1 Bacteriology and pathophysiology of *H. pylori*

The bacteria that is responsible for infection of the stomach was originally noted as an incidental finding on many gastric biopsies. Further speciation of bacteria found that it was related to campylobacter. It was later further defined and speciated and renamed to be *Helicobacter pylori*.

H. pylori is a spiral shaped, gram-negative bacterium that can be cultured on blood agar or selective media (Skirrow's) [3]. This bacterium is catalase, oxidase and urease positive. Urease positivity is both vital to the organism's survival and clinically relevant as it is the basis of several diagnostic assays.

There are several inherent factors that ensure survival in a hostile environment within the gastric mucosa including urease activity, motility, and the ability to adhere to gastric epithelial lining [4].

Bacterial urease hydrolyzes gastric urea to form ammonia, which facilitates invasion of the gastric mucus layer via neutralization of the acidic protective layer of the stomach [5]. The unique morphology of the spiral shaped bacterium and flagellated motility contribute to the ability to adhere to gastric mucosa. *H. pylori* attaches to gastric epithelium via receptor-mediated adhesion. Susceptibility of the host is multifactorial and dependent on cellular expression of surface receptors, which renders some individuals more susceptible to penetration and colonization leading to pathologic response. In summation, the four steps necessary for successful colonization described by Kao et al. are survival in the acidic environment, movement toward epithelium via flagella motility, attachment to host cells by adhesin-receptor interactions, and tissue damage by bacterial toxin release [6].

3. Indications for testing

The established indications for testing patients for *H. pylori* include gastric marginal zone lymphoma of mucosa associated lymphoid tissue, active peptic ulcer disease or history of peptic ulcer if the cure of *H. pylori* infection has not been documented, and early gastric cancer [7].

If any of the following are identified on endoscopic evaluation: actively bleeding peptic ulcer, other endoscopic abnormality requiring gastric biopsy, or a clinical history of proton pumping inhibitor, bismuth, or antibiotic use warrant biopsy for *H. pylori* testing. Endoscopy is not indicated for the sole purpose of establishing a diagnosis of *H. pylori* infection. Other indications for *H. pylori* that are more controversial include uninvestigated dyspepsia and patients less than 60 years of age without alarm features, chronic treatment with non-steroidal anti-inflammatory drugs or aspirin, unexplained iron deficiency [8], and adults with immune thrombocytopenia [9].

Medications that should be discontinued prior to *H. pylori* testing include proton pump inhibitors as well as bismuth and antibiotics. Proton pump inhibitors within one to 2 weeks can decrease sensitivity of all endoscopic based testing as well as non-invasive testing. Antibiotics and bismuth within 2–4 weeks of testing also decreases sensitivity. Patients should be advised to stop proton pump inhibitors one to 2 weeks prior to testing if feasible testing should be performed at least 4 weeks after completion of any bismuth and antibiotic treatment [7]. Stool antigen testing and urea breath testing are appropriate for people who do not otherwise require endoscopy.

3.1 Methods of noninvasive diagnosis—Urea breath and stool antigen assay, serology

Of the myriad diagnostic tests available, all with various ranges of sensitivity and specificity, there is not one single test that can be considered a gold standard. Typically, a combination of invasive and noninvasive tests can lead to an accurate diagnosis. One of the notable disadvantages of invasive testing is the requirements of tertiary laboratory equipment and staff. Thus, several noninvasive tests have been developed.

3.1.1 Urea breath testing (UBT)

The basis of UBT involves the bacterium urease mechanism of action. Urease enzyme hydrolyzes urea within the gastric lumen to produce carbon dioxide and ammonia. The assay involves ingestion of urea with a carbon labeled isotope (typically, nonradioactive 13C or radioactive 14C). In afflicted individuals, *H. pylori* releases the labeled CO2, which is detected in breath samples. The test can be performed with relative ease and within 15–20 minutes. The sensitivity and specificity of UBT are greater than 95% [10]. False-positive results are uncommon; however, false negative results are seen in patients with recent PPI and antibiotic use. Additionally special equipment is required for the test which can limit its clinical use in areas of limited resources.

3.1.2 Stool antigen testing

The presence of bacterial antigen within stool samples is indicative of an ongoing age pylori infection. Thus, stool antigen testing can be used to diagnose and confirm *H. pylori* infection as well as confirm eradication. The sensitivity and specificity of stool antigen testing is comparable to that of urea breath testing at greater than 95%. Additionally, stool antigen testing can be affected by recent PP, bismuth, and antibiotic use. A limitation of stool antigen testing not seen in UBT is a patient reluctance to give stool samples. Of the available noninvasive testing, stool antigen testing is the most cost effective in areas of limited resources as well as intermediate prevalence *H. pylori* infection [11].

3.1.3 Serology

ELISA test to detect immunoglobulin G antibodies generated against *H. pylori* is both inexpensive and noninvasive. This method requires reliable laboratory staffing with appropriate controls and can be impractical in routine practice. In areas with low prevalence populations and limited resources and limited resources can lead to inaccurate serologic testing results. While the sensitivity is greater than 95, specificity has been reported as low as 60% [12]. Another limitation of this method is the failure of it to distinguish between active and past infection.

3.2 Invasive methods of diagnosis

Endoscopy is the basis for invasive methods of diagnosing *H. pylori*. Tissue biopsies are used to perform several assays including urease testing, culture, and histologic examination to determine presence of *H. pylori* organisms. The ideal location of biopsy has been studied, both antral and fundal biopsies have been determined to yield the most accurate diagnosis. Incisura angularis biopsies are not recommended as they have been shown to have the lowest yield of positive diagnosis [13–15].

3.2.1 Histology

Historically, histologic evaluation of gastric mucosa was the first method of accurate diagnosis of *H. pylori* infection. The presence of the unique spiral shaped bacteria along with inflammatory changes within the mucosa on microscopic evaluation is considered a positive diagnosis [16]. A multitude of stains, including Giemsa, Hp silver stain, and immunostaining have been used to detect *H. pylori*. Hematoxylin and eosin stains help to evaluate the extent of inflammatory changes as well as with the detection of the bacteria [17]. Since its discovery, more complex histologic examination techniques have been employed in the microscopic evaluation of *H. pylori*. Genta stain, a combination of three commonly available stains (Steiner, hematoxylin-eosin, and alcian blue) is particularly advantageous as it visualizes both inflammatory changes and *H. pylori* [18]. Typically, the routine use of Giemsa stain is a simple, highly sensitive and cost-effective method of histologic diagnosis of *H. pylori* infection.

The Sydney System of classification of gastritis was originally described in 1996 and has had multiple revisions since its inception. The Sydney system classifies the severity of gastritis by the following histologic findings: the extent of lymphocyte and neutrophil invasion and the lamina propria, glandular atrophy within the corpus and antrum, intestinal metaplasia of the mucosal epithelium, and the amount of *H. pylori* organisms present (**Figure 1**) [19].

3.2.2 Rapid urease test (RUT)

Rapid Urease test (RUT) is another invasive method of detection of *H. pylori* infection. The basis of the test revolves around the ability of *H. pylori* bacteria to

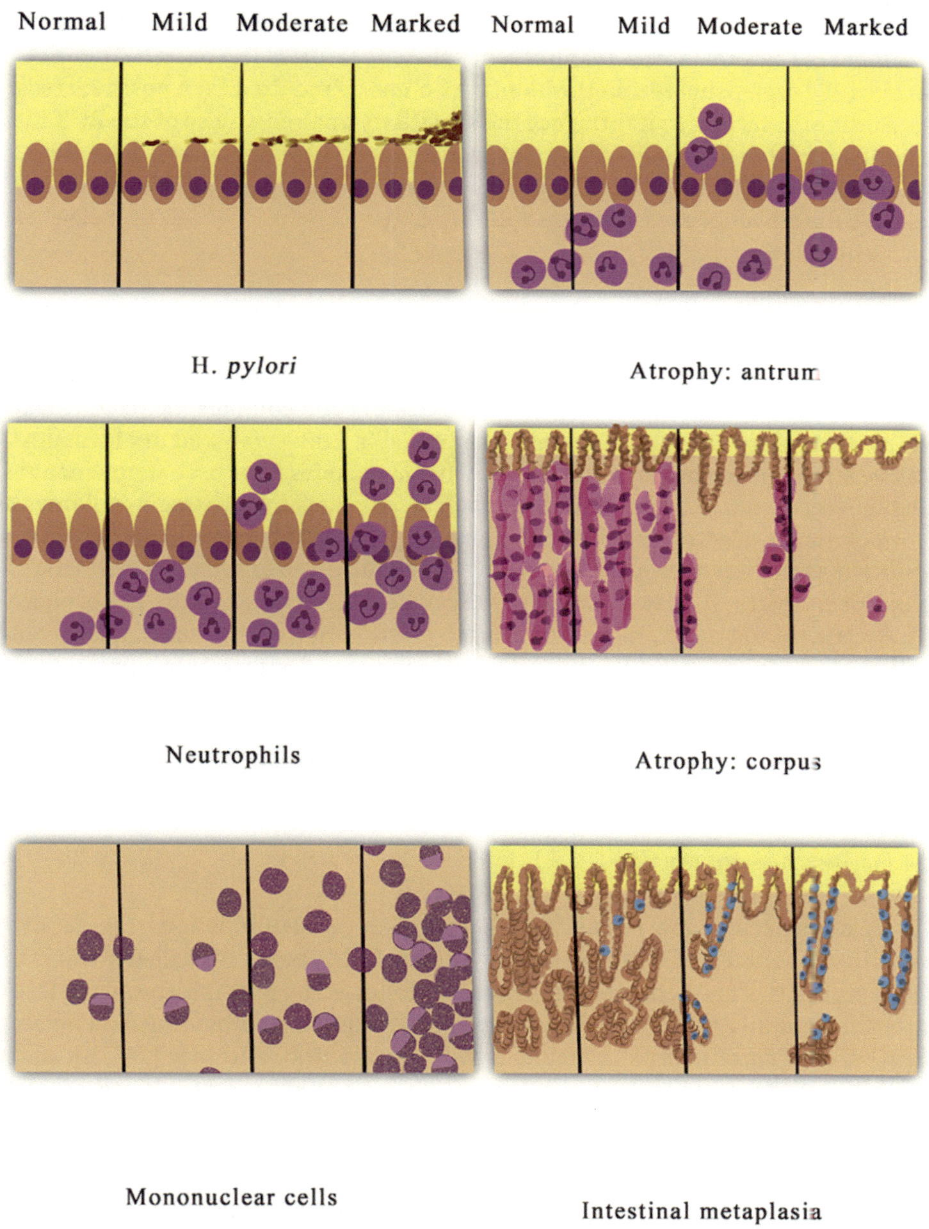

Figure 1.
Grading of gastritis by Sydney system: acute inflammation, chronic inflammation, atrophic gastritis, intestinal metaplasia, and Helicobacter pylori *density.*

convert urea into carbon dioxide and ammonia. Once the biopsy is obtained, it is placed within a test container. Once the *H. pylori* within the specimen splits the urea to ammonia, the elevation of pH by ammonium hydroxide is detected by pH indicator color change. Tests can be performed either in solution or a solid supporting medium [20]. The Campylobacter-like organism (CLO) test is a commercially available kit that contains solid media, and typically takes up to 24 hours to result. The Pyloritek kit utilizes a reagent strip for the rapid urease test where a positive result can be obtained within 1 hour. Both kits have similar sensitivity and specificity; however, the Pyloritek kits are more convenient for use in endoscopy clinics given rapidity of results [21].

It is notable that while both kits have sensitivity and specificity greater than 90%, there are several factors that influence these measures. The bacterial density of at least 10^4 organisms within the biopsy specimen is required for a positive result [22]. Additional factors that influence the specificity and sensitivity of the RUT kits include bacterial density post-treatment, patients with bleeding ulcers at the time of biopsy, patients taking H2-receptor antagonists or PPIs [23, 24]. Urease testing does have the advantage over culture and histology given the low cost, user ease, and rapidity of results.

3.2.3 Culture

H. pylori can be isolated by culture from gastric biopsy samples. The microbe requires a hypercapnic, microaerophilic environment and complex media for isolation [3]. Following biopsy, samples must be placed in saline vials and not formalin for successful culture and analysis. Typical media includes Agar base supplemented with blood or serum. Various antibiotics such as vancomycin, bacitracin, polymyxin, are often used in selective media for *H. pylori* [25]. Isolated bacteria grow best in a humid atmosphere at a temperature of 37C and require five to 7 days of incubation. For optimal growth, 5–10% carbon dioxide can be added to the culture atmosphere [26]. Because of the patchy distribution of *H. pylori* within the stomach, it is recommended to take biopsies 2 cm proximal to the pylorus and at least two biopsies from the anterior and posterior corpus [27]. Culture is not considered first line testing for establishing a diagnosis of *H. pylori* because it is time-consuming and often tedious; however, culture data allows for testing of antibiotic sensitivity to choose appropriate antibiotic regimen for eradication.

3.2.4 Polymerase chain reaction (PCR)

PCR is a molecular analysis method that involves rapid production of copies of a specific segment of DNA. It uses short synthetic DNA fragments called primers to select a segment of the genome to be amplified followed by multiple rounds of DNA synthesis to amplify the segment of interest. PCR is useful in providing data involving the presence of certain virulent factors as well as antibiotic resistance [26]. An advantage of PCR is that a variety of clinical samples can be used to extract *H. pylori* DNA including gastric biopsy, gastric secretions, saliva, dental plaque, and stool samples; therefore, it can be utilized for both invasive and non-invasive diagnosis. When utilizing stool samples for PCR assay, a separate extraction step must be performed to separate the *H. pylori* DNA from the stool sample, as it typically contains a variety of commensal bacteria and PCR-inhibiting chemicals that may lead to false-negative and false-positive results [28]. PCR stool testing is advantageous as the patient needs to provide only a small sample (usually 50–200 mg) of fresh stool sample, and results can be obtained within hours of sample submission, facilitating treatment decisions in real time [28]. The overall cost of fecal PCR testing is lower than invasive methods, negating the need for the expense of hospital admission and anesthesia.

Antibiotic resistance is one of the leading causes of failure of treatment of *H. pylori*. Specific gene identification can be used for both bacterial detection and lend information regarding antibiotic resistance, notably, the 23S rRNA gene. Specific point mutations within this gene can lead to clarithromycin resistance [29]. Other genes that have been identified that confer antibiotic resistance include rdxA/frxA with metronidazole resistance [30, 31], 16S ribosomal DNA with tetracycline resistance [32], and gyrA gene in fluoroquinolone resistance [33]. PCR based testing has a significant role in both non-invasive and invasive methods of diagnosis of *H. pylori* and can guide effective treatment.

4. Conclusions

There is no one gold standard test that is recommended for a diagnosis of *H. pylori* infection. Of the non-invasive tests discussed, each has their distinct advantages and disadvantages as well as varied sensitivity and specificity. Invasive testing across the board has higher sensitivity and specificity, but requires biopsy, which may not be indicated in certain patient populations for initial screening for *H. pylori* infection. A combination of one non-invasive and invasive test tends to be the overall recommended gold standard for accurate diagnosis of *H. pylori*.

Author details

Taylor Fontenot and Annabel E. Barber*
Kirk Kerkorian School of Medicine at UNLV, Las Vegas, NV, USA

*Address all correspondence to: annabel.barber@unlv.edu

References

[1] Brown LM. *Helicobacter pylori*: Epidemiology and routes of transmission. Epidemiologic Reviews. 2000;**22**(2):283-297. DOI: 10.1093/oxfordjournals.epirev.a018040

[2] Marshall BJ, Warren JR. Unidentified curved bacilli in the stomach of patients with gastritis and peptic ulceration. Lancet. 1984;**1**(8390):1311-1315. DOI: 10.1016/s0140-6736(84)91816-6

[3] Goodwin CS, Worsley BW. Microbiology of *helicobacter pylori*. Gastroenterology Clinics of North America. 1993;**22**(1):5-19

[4] Amieva MR, El-Omar EM. Host-bacterial interactions in *helicobacter pylori* infection. Gastroenterology. 2008;**134**(1):306-323. DOI: 10.1053/j.gastro.2007.11.009

[5] Mobley HL. The role of *helicobacter pylori* urease in the pathogenesis of gastritis and peptic ulceration. Alimentary Pharmacology & Therapeutics. 1996;**10**(Suppl. 1):57-64. DOI:10.1046/j.1365-2036.1996.22164006.x

[6] Kao CY, Sheu BS, Wu JJ. *Helicobacter pylori* infection: An overview of bacterial virulence factors and pathogenesis. Biomedical Journal. 2016;**39**(1):14-23

[7] Malfertheiner P, Megraud F, O'Morain CA, Atherton J, Axon AT, Bazzoli F, et al. Management of *Helicobacter pylori* infection--the Maastricht IV/ Florence consensus report. Gut. 2012;**61**(5):646-664. DOI: 10.1136/gutjnl-2012-302084

[8] DuBois S, Kearney DJ. Iron-deficiency anemia and *helicobacter pylori* infection: A review of the evidence. The American Journal of Gastroenterology. 2005;**100**(2):453-459. DOI: 10.1111/j.1572-0241.2005.30252.x

[9] Rostami N, Keshtkar-Jahromi M, Rahnavardi M, Keshtkar-Jahromi M, Esfahani FS. Effect of eradication of *helicobacter pylori* on platelet recovery in patients with chronic idiopathic thrombocytopenic purpura: A controlled trial. American Journal of Hematology. 2008;**83**(5):376-381. DOI: 10.1002/ajh.21125

[10] Howden CW, Hunt RH. Guidelines for the management of *helicobacter pylori* infection. Ad hoc committee on practice parameters of the American College of Gastroenterology. The American Journal of Gastroenterology. 1998;**93**(12):2330-2338. DOI: 10.1111/j.1572-0241.1998.00684.x

[11] Vakil N, Rhew D, Soll A, Ofman JJ. The cost-effectiveness of diagnostic testing strategies for *helicobacter pylori*. The American Journal of Gastroenterology. 2000;**95**(7):1691-1698. DOI: 10.1111/j.1572-0241.2000.02193.x

[12] Chey WD, Wong BC. Practice parameters Committee of the American College of gastroenterology. American College of Gastroenterology guideline on the management of *helicobacter pylori* infection. The American Journal of Gastroenterology. 2007;**102**(8):1808-1825. DOI: 10.1111/j.1572-0241.2007.01393.x. Epub 2007 Jun 29

[13] Patel SK, Pratap CB, Jain AK, Gulati AK, Nath G. Diagnosis of *helicobacter pylori*: What should be the gold standard? World Journal of Gastroenterology. 2014;**20**(36):12847-12859. DOI: 10.3748/wjg.v20.i36.12847

[14] Lash JG, Genta RM. Adherence to the Sydney system guidelines increases the detection of helicobacter gastritis and intestinal metaplasia in 400738 sets of gastric biopsies. Alimentary Pharmacology & Therapeutics. 2013;**38**:424-431. DOI: 10.1111/apt.12383

[15] Lopes AI, Vale FF, Oleastro M. *Helicobacter pylori* infection—Recent developments in diagnosis. World Journal of Gastroenterology. 2014;**20**(28):9299-9313. DOI: 10.3748/wjg.v20.i28.9299

[16] Rotimi O, Cairns A, Gray S, Moayyedi P, Dixon MF. Histological identification of *helicobacter pylori*: Comparison of staining methods. Journal of Clinical Pathology. 2000;**53**:756-759

[17] Laine L, Lewin DN, Naritoku W, Cohen H. Prospective comparison of H&E, Giemsa, and Genta stains for the diagnosis of *helicobacter pylori*. Gastrointestinal Endoscopy. 1997;**45**:463-467

[18] Genta RM, Robason GO, Graham DY. Simultaneous visualization of *helicobacter pylori* and gastric morphology: A new stain. Human Pathology. 1994;**25**(3):221-226. DOI: 10.1016/0046-8177(94)90191-0

[19] Stolte M, Meining A. The updated Sydney system: Classification and grading of gastritis as the basis of diagnosis and treatment. Canadian Journal of Gastroenterology. 2001;**15**(9):591-598. DOI: 10.1155/2001/367832

[20] Kato M, Shimizu Y, Kobayashi T, Komatsu Y, Takeda H, Sugiyama T, et al. Rapid urease test. Nihon Rinsho. 2003;**61**(1):72-78 Japanese

[21] Mcnicholl AG, Ducons J, et al. *Helicobacter pylori* study Group of the Asociación Española de Gastroenterología (AEG). Accuracy of the ultra-rapid urease test for diagnosis of *helicobacter pylori* infection. Gastroenterología y Hepatología. 2017;**40**(10):651-657. English, Spanish. DOI: 10.1016/j.gastrohep.2017.07.007

[22] Puetz T, Vakil N, Phadnis S, Dunn B, Robinson J. The Pyloritek test and the CLO test: Accuracy and incremental cost analysis. The American Journal of Gastroenterology. 1997;**92**(2):254-257

[23] Mégraud F. Advantages and disadvantages of current diagnostic tests for the detection of *helicobacter pylori*. Scandinavian Journal of Gastroenterology. Supplement. 1996;**215**:57-62. DOI: 10.3109/00365529609094536

[24] Lerang F, Moum B, Mowinckel P, Haug JB, Ragnhildstveit E, Berge T, et al. Accuracy of seven different tests for the diagnosis of *helicobacter pylori* infection and the impact of H2-receptor antagonists on test results. Scandinavian Journal of Gastroenterology. 1998;**33**(4):364-369. DOI: 10.1080/00365529850170982

[25] Mégraud F, Lehours P. *Helicobacter pylori* detection and antimicrobial susceptibility testing. Clinical Microbiology Reviews. 2007;**20**:280-322

[26] Saez J, Belda S, Santibáñez M, Rodríguez JC, Sola-Vera J, Galiana A, et al. Real-time PCR for diagnosing *helicobacter pylori* infection in patients with upper gastrointestinal bleeding: Comparison with other classical diagnostic methods. Journal of Clinical Microbiology. 2012;**50**:3233-3323

[27] Cover TL. Perspectives on methodology for in vitro culture of *helicobacter pylori*. Methods in Molecular Biology. 2012;**921**:11-15. DOI: 10.1007/978-1-62703-005-2_3

[28] Rimbara E, Sasatsu M, Graham DY. PCR detection of *helicobacter pylori* in clinical samples. Methods in Molecular Biology. 2013;**943**:279-287. DOI: 10.1007/978-1-60327-353-4_19

[29] Gong RJ, Xu CX, Li H, Liu XM. Polymerase chain reaction-based tests for detecting *helicobacter pylori* clarithromycin resistance in stool samples: A meta-analysis. World Journal of Clinical Cases. 2021;**9**(1):133-147. DOI: 10.12998/wjcc.v9.i1.133

[30] Kwon DH, Kato M, El-Zaatari FA, Osato MS, Graham DY. Frame-shift mutations in NAD(P)H flavin oxidoreductase encoding gene (frxA) from metronidazole resistant *helicobacter pylori* ATCC43504 and its involvement in metronidazole resistance. FEMS Microbiology Letters. 2000;**188**:197-202

[31] Jenks PJ, Ferrero RL, Labigne A. The role of the rdxA gene in the evolution of metronidazole resistance in *helicobacter pylori*. The Journal of Antimicrobial Chemotherapy. 1999;**43**:753-758

[32] Dailidiene D, Bertoli MT, Miciuleviciene J, Mukhopadhyay AK, Dailide G, Pascasio MA, et al. Emergence of tetracycline resistance in *helicobacter pylori*: Multiple mutational changes in 16S ribosomal DNA and other genetic loci. Antimicrobial Agents and Chemotherapy. 2002;**46**:3940-3946

[33] Moore RA, Beckthold B, Wong S, Kureishi A, Bryan LE. Nucleotide sequence of the gyrA gene and characterization of ciprofloxacin-resistant mutants of *helicobacter pylori*. Antimicrobial Agents and Chemotherapy. 1995;**39**:107-111

Chapter 4

Linked Color Imaging in Endoscopic Diagnosis for *Helicobacter pylori*

Yu Chen and Weiguang Qiao

Abstract

Linked color imaging (LCI), distinct from the traditional red emphasis in endoscopic imaging, utilizes narrow-band light and red signal processing to enhance contrast in mucosal color. Redness and erosion triggered by inflammation are recognized as typical signs of *Helicobacter pylori* (HP) infection. Notably, these visual cues are readily identifiable through the LCI mode. Leveraging the LCI observation mode significantly improves the accuracy of diagnosing gastritis associated with HP, providing accurate diagnostic performance and precise localization. LCI demonstrates superior diagnostic accuracy in detecting HP infections, including their precise localization, when compared to traditional white light endoscopy. It also holds promise for enhancing the precision of sampling for HP cultures and determining antibiotic susceptibility. Integrating LCI with the Kyoto Classification of Gastritis may enhance the endoscopic diagnosis and confirmation of HP infection eradication, subsequently augmenting the capacity of gastrointestinal endoscopists and general practitioners to identify HP infections through endoscopic imagery.

Keywords: linked color imaging, image-enhancing endoscopy, *Helicobacter pylori*, accuracy, targeted biopsies, artificial intelligence, education

1. Introduction

In recent times, progress in image-enhancing endoscopy (IEE) has significantly enhanced the capacity to identify and diagnose gastric cancer in its early stages. Methods encompassed by IEE, such as narrow band imaging (NBI), blue laser imaging (BLI), and linked color imaging (LCI) [1], are instrumental in advancing this field. Particularly, LCI, as a distinct mode within the blue-laser endoscopy framework, intensifies the contrast of red hues relative to the surrounding area by adjusting the light components' intensity and mix [2]. In LCI, post-processing boosts brightness and color contrast, making it well-suited for distant views. This enhancement allows red areas to appear more vividly red and white areas to appear whiter, facilitating the identification of suspicious lesions by endoscopists. A key feature of LCI is its ability to provide images with enhanced color differences (CD), aiding in the differentiation of suspicious lesions from the surrounding mucosa based on color. Studies have reported that the demarcation of lesions in LCI mode is clearer than that in white light imaging (WLI) mode [3].

LCI effectively distinguishes early gastric cancer (EGC) as orange-red and intestinal metaplasia as purple, regardless of *Helicobacter pylori* (HP) eradication history. It significantly aids in the detection of superficial EGC. Additionally, LCI is pivotal in determining HP infection status, closely linked with gastric cancer risk. Utilizing trans-nasal (ultra-thin) endoscopy with LCI proves beneficial in identifying gastric neoplastic lesions. Recent prospective studies highlight LCI's superior detection rate for gastric cancer compared to WLI. We advocate for the integration of LCI into standard upper gastrointestinal endoscopies to enhance early detection and diagnosis [4].

Real-time endoscopy is crucial for diagnosing HP infection and facilitating targeted biopsy [5]. In clinical practice, real-time endoscopy in conjunction with conventional WLI and IEE techniques, such as NBI, LCI, and BLI, plays a significant role in identifying HP-infected status [6]. Compared to conventional WLI, LCI has been demonstrated to aid in determining HP infection status, a factor closely linked to the risk of developing gastric cancer. Additionally, LCI offers enhanced detection of gastric cancer, owing to its superior color differentiation when compared to adjacent tissues. This improvement enhances lesion detection in distant views and facilitates the more accurate diagnosis of gastric neoplasms.

2. LCI character of HP state

The presence of HP is commonly associated with increased susceptibility to gastric cancer, a condition often preceded by chronic gastritis, marked atrophy of the gastric mucosa, and intestinal metaplasia [7]. During endoscopic stomach screenings, it is vital to categorize gastritis into three phases: never-infected, currently-infected, and previously-infected, which also includes an after-eradication phase. Retrospective studies conducted in Japan have shown that LCI is superior to WLI in accurately identifying HP-positive mucosa, boasting a sensitivity of 93.3% and a specificity of 78.3% [8]. Therefore, LCI appears to play a crucial role in determining the status of HP infections.

2.1 HP-uninfected mucosa

HP-negative mucosa after eradication is distinctly observed as apricot in color (**Figure 1A** and **B**). The adjacent mucosal tissue uniformly presented a pale orange hue, reminiscent of a white-apricot blend, in all areas containing fundic glands. It's noteworthy that the color characteristics of gastric lesions may be affected by the absorption of violet light at 410 nm within the superficial layer of the mucosa [8].

2.2 HP-infected mucosa

In LCI imaging, the widespread redness seen in the gastric mucosa of the gastric body, a hallmark sign of present HP infection, appears distinctly as a deep crimson color (**Figure 1C–P**) [9], while intestinal metaplasia appears clearly as lavender (**Figure 1I** and **J** arrowheads). Regarding LCI visuals, the indication of HP infection is identified by any of these criteria: (1) widespread reddening; (2) absence of a regular arrangement of collecting venules (RAC); and (3) adherence of mucus [10].

A study conducted a correlation analysis to assess the indicators associated with HP infection. Based on the findings of skilled endoscopists, there was a notable association between HP infection and several indicators: WLI and LCI scores, the

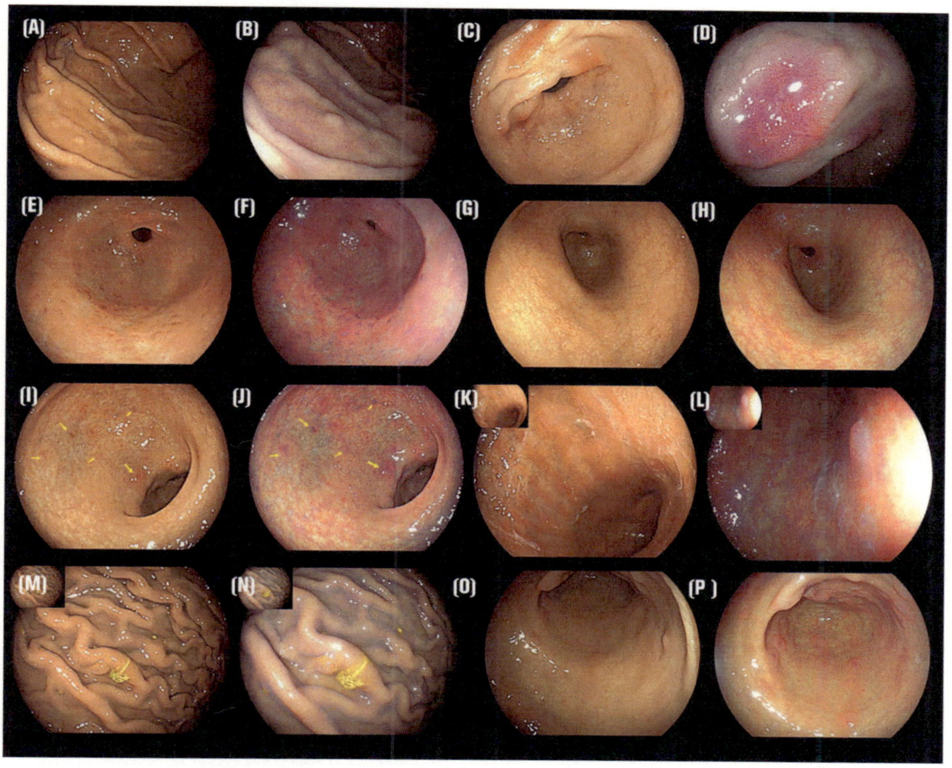

Figure 1.
Endoscopic schematic diagram: (A) WLI of RAC (+) with HP uninfected, (B) LCI of RAC (+) with HP uninfected, (C) WLI of diffuse redness, (D) LCI of diffuse redness, (E) WLI of map-like redness, (F) LCI of map-like redness, (G) WLI of nodular gastritis, (H) LCI of nodular gastritis, (I) WLI of atrophic gastritis (type C) and intestinal metaplasia (arrowheads), (J) LCI of atrophic gastritis (type C) and intestinal metaplasia (arrowheads), (K) WLI of atrophic gastritis (type O), (L) LCI of atrophic gastritis (type O), (M) WLI of rugal hypertrophy and fundie gland polyps, (N) LCI of rugal hypertrophy and fundic gland polyps, (O) WLI of red streak, (P) LCI of red streak.

reddening and purpleness of the fundic gland mucosa, and the cloudiness of the mucus lake [11]. In contrast, granular erosion, erythema, and loss of collecting venules were moderately correlated with HP. According to Dohi et al., LCI enhanced the endoscopic diagnosis of active HP infections, demonstrating improvements of 10–15% in accuracy, sensitivity, and specificity compared to WLI [8]. The rate of diagnosis using the LCI method for HP infection surpassed that of other methods.

LCI may serve as an effective preliminary diagnostic instrument for HP infections in real-time applications, offering a notable level of diagnostic precision. Shida et al. concluded that LED endoscopy is equivalent to laser endoscopy for assessing HP infection status [12].

In a prospective study, the distinction in hue at the degenerated margins was markedly more pronounced using LCI than WLI, irrespective of the HP infection status. LCI exhibited a notable enhancement in diagnostic precision for subjects with either a current or historical HP infection, as opposed to WLI. Conversely, in prospective diagnostic research focusing on HP infection, the diagnostic precision, sensitivity, and specificity metrics for WLI, LCI, and magnified endoscopy using WLI, when evaluating the presence of RAC or general erythema, did not present considerable variances [13].

2.3 HP-eradicated mucosa

After eradication, HP-negative mucosa is distinctly observed as apricot in color. However, a considerable amount of red depression is evident extensively throughout the gastric mucosa, spanning from the gastric body to the antrum. It has been observed that through the application of LCI technology, the mucosa of the fundic gland exhibits widespread redness (resembling a deep shade of crimson) in cases of active gastritis, whereas it manifests a pale orange hue (akin to the shade of white apricots) in stomachs where HP has been successfully eradicated [14]. Majima et al. found that LCI detects the positive risk indicator of map-like redness (MR) (**Figure 1E** and **F**). The negative risk indicator of a regular arrangement of collecting venules for early gastric cancer (EGC) detection after HP eradication is more frequent than WLI [15]. LCI was more efficient for evaluating MR than WLI because LCI could identify MR more frequently than WLI. Hence, it might be tentatively inferred that the influence of external variables on the LCI mode was relatively minimal regarding the diagnosis of HP. The study revealed that when reviewing recorded endoscopies, both expert and trainee endoscopists had a notably reduced miss rate for EGC post-eradication when using LCI compared to WLI. Concerning the objective analyses, it evaluated the CD of each lesion on WLI and LCI images [16].

2.4 The meta-analysis and limitation

To thoroughly assess the diagnostic efficacy of LCI and WLI in detecting HP infection, we conducted a meta-analysis. It employs a meticulously crafted framework of study inclusion criteria, ensuring a high standard of selection precision. In conducting this analysis, we rigorously adhered to a set of carefully pre-established criteria for selecting relevant studies. Included studies were either randomized controlled trials or observational studies, aimed at comparing the sensitivity and specificity of LCI versus WLI in detecting HP infection. The investigation entailed systematic searches within the PubMed and CNKI databases, utilizing key phrases including "((Linked Color Imaging) AND (White Light Imaging)) AND (*Helicobacter pylori* Infection)" among others. Studies were excluded if they were published in languages other than English or Chinese, were case reports or review articles, or if they contained incomplete data. For each study included in the analysis, details such as the author's name, year of publication, design of the study, number of participants, and sensitivity and specificity outcomes for both LCI and WLI were meticulously gathered. This data extraction was performed independently by two researchers, with any discrepancies resolved by a third.

We employed the QUADAS-2 framework for evaluating the quality of the studies we included, focusing on the bias risk and relevance in aspects such as patient selection, index tests, reference standards, flow, and timing. Based on these parameters, each study was classified as a "low," "high," or "unclear" risk. In our meta-analysis, most studies were deemed low risk in patient selection and index tests, but some showed moderate risk in flow and timing (**Figure 2**).

The meta-analysis results, synthesized through a random-effects model, demonstrated LCI's superior sensitivity (91%) and specificity (88%) in detecting HP infection. This contrasts with WLI's sensitivity and specificity, which stood at 82% and 80%, respectively. Our heterogeneity assessment revealed I^2 values of 45% for sensitivity and 50% for specificity, indicating moderate variability across studies. Nonetheless, the observed P-value of 0.07 from the chi-square test indicated that the existing

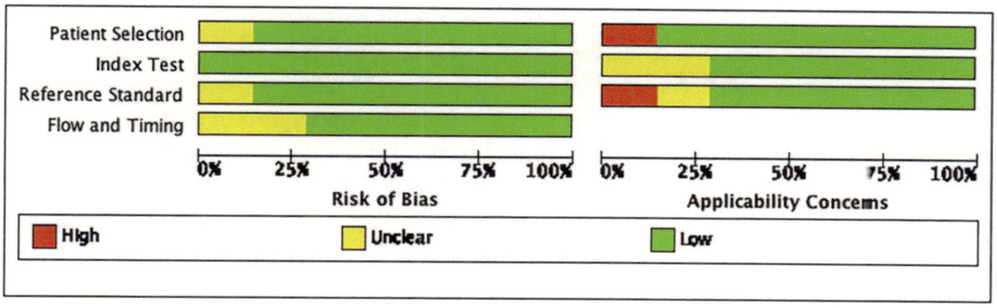

Figure 2.
Assessment of study quality using QUADAS-2 tool presents bar graphs depicting the risk of bias and applicability concerns in various studies. The majority of included randomized controlled trials (RCTs) demonstrated a low risk in patient selection and index testing (axes: horizontal axis: proportion (%) ranging from 0% to 100%, vertical axis: aspects of study quality assessment: patient selection, index tests, reference standards, flow and timing, color legend: red: high risk, yellow: unclear risk, green: low risk).

heterogeneity was not of statistical significance, suggesting that the variations across individual studies were not substantial enough to notably influence the aggregate outcome. Further strengthening LCI's diagnostic value, summary receiver operating characteristic (SROC) analysis showed an area under the curve (AUC) of 0.94, underscoring LCI's efficacy and accuracy in diagnosing HP infection. In contrast, WLI's AUC was 0.88, slightly lagging in diagnostic performance (**Figure 3**).

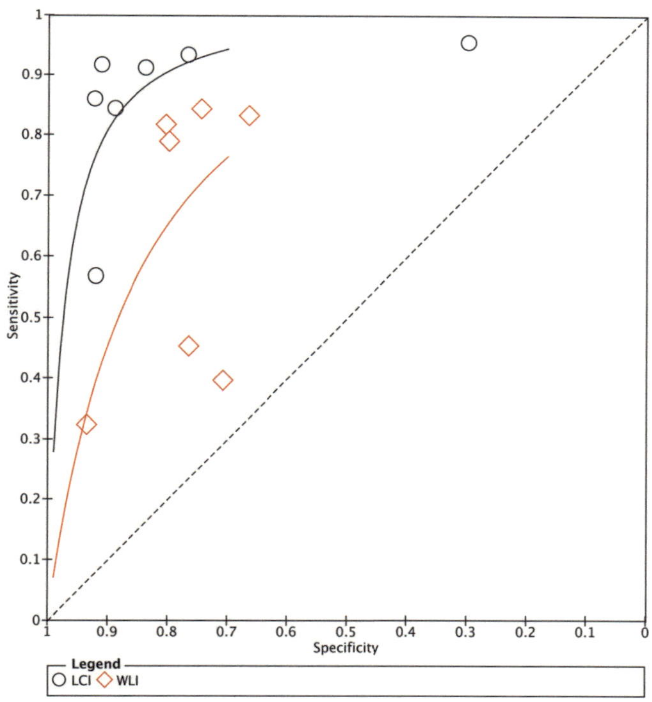

Figure 3.
SROC curve comparison: LCI vs. WLI. LCI demonstrates superior efficacy over WLI in HP detection. This figure compares the receiver operating characteristic (ROC) curves of LCI and WLI for detecting HP infection. The x-axis is "1-specificity" (false-positive rate), and the y-axis is sensitivity (true-positive rate). LCI data points are represented by hollow circles and WLI data points by hollow diamonds. The AUC reflects test accuracy, with higher values indicating better sensitivity and specificity. LCI demonstrates superior efficacy over WLI in HP detection.

In instances of pronounced atrophy, the hue alterations post-HP infection tend to be inconspicuous, resulting in a lack of widespread redness when observed using LCI technology. The negative predictive value (NPV) of RAC exhibits optimal performance, in contrast, the positive predictive value (PPV) is notably inadequate. Furthermore, the morphological attributes exhibit variations throughout the different phases of atrophic evolution [17]. Since various endoscopic characteristics must be comprehensively assessed for an accurate endoscopic diagnosis, inter-observer bias exists in the studies.

In summary, LCI demonstrates a clear advantage in diagnosing HP infection. Its high sensitivity and specificity, coupled with superior overall diagnostic efficacy, render LCI a more valuable diagnostic tool. Despite some heterogeneity among studies, LCI's overall performance stands out, offering robust technological support for clinical diagnosis.

3. LCI for screening early gastric cancer

Moreover, the diverse coloration present in the surrounding mucosal tissue raises debates regarding whether color intensification aids in identifying EGC. In the context of WLI, the endoscopic visuals of these observations closely mimic cancerous appearances, making the differentiation between non-malignant and malignant growths challenging. In contrast, gastric cancer is recognized as orange or magenta, while surrounding lesions are observed in lavender color in LCI, allowing for clearer observation compared to WLI due to enhanced color contrast [16]. The presence of intestinal metaplasia is characterized by a distinct lavender coloration. Because of these prominent color disparities, research indicates that LCI has a markedly superior detection rate for intestinal metaplasia compared to WLI [18]. Additionally, a study conducted by Ono et al. further supported that the lavender hue observed in LCI facilitates the non-invasive identification of gastrointestinal metaplasia [19]. MR was identified more frequently using LCI than WLI, and the absence of RAC was associated with the detection of EGC after the eradication of HP [15]. LCI had the highest visibility among findings of gastric mucosa and EGC after HP eradication. A recent meta-analysis demonstrated that LCI exhibits strong diagnostic efficacy for gastrointestinal metaplasia [20]. Additionally, when examined using LCI, the vascular permeation of the atrophic border and the atrophic region becomes more discernible compared to observations made with WLI [21]. It has also been documented that endoscopic procedures utilizing LED for LCI are proficient in the early identification of EGC [22]. The color difference value with LCI was significantly higher, being more than twice that of WLI, and this difference appeared to be similar in cases of accompanying HP infection or intestinal metaplasia. However, no statistically significant finding was present in signet ring cell carcinoma or mixed-type histology [23].

3.1 EGC strategy

3.1.1 HP-related gastritis

The LCI score has been shown to exhibit notable sensitivity and specificity in distinguishing HP-associated gastritis. This underscores its efficacy as a method for detecting HP presence in gastric mucosal tissue [24]. In an investigation, both erythema and non-visible RAC were incorporated into the regression analysis, proving beneficial for distinguishing HP-induced gastritis. Conversely, features like erosions and nodularity were excluded from this model [11]. Mizukami et al.'s research indicated that LCI enhanced the definition of the atrophic border through objective analysis [21]. In a multicenter prospective study conducted by Ono et al., which compared the accuracy of WLI and LCI for the endoscopic diagnosis of HP gastritis, LCI exhibited notably superior performance over WLI, particularly in patients with a history of past infections [25]. LED-LCI was found to be more effective than WLI for evaluating HP-related gastritis. However, another study suggested no significant differences in accuracy, sensitivity, or specificity for diagnosing metaplastic gastritis between LCI and WLI [26].

3.1.2 MESDA-G

The Magnifying Endoscopy Simple Diagnostic Algorithm for Early Gastric Cancer (MESDA-G) provides an extensive framework for the early detection of gastric cancer. It evaluates the boundary differentiation between abnormal lesions and normal gastric tissue, as well as identifies anomalies in the microvascular structure and surface patterns of the stomach lining [27]. Given that most gastric cancers are enveloped by intestinal metaplasia, LCI proves valuable in depicting this metaplasia in pale purple. The majority of the surrounding mucosa is also represented in purple, creating a high color contrast. In the LCI view, early-stage gastric cancers typically appear orange-red, orange, or orange-white [1]. It becomes crucial to identify gastric cancer (depicted in orange) amidst intestinal epithelial metaplasia (depicted in purple) using LCI. Subsequent clarification of the diagnosis can be achieved through magnifying BLI. LCI has proven to be effective in the early detection of flat gastric cancers, manifesting as distinct reddish lesions against the surrounding mucosa [28]. In the LCI view, undifferentiated gastric cancer exhibits a faded tone, characteristic of mucosa in HP-uninfected cases, offering clear color differentiation [2]. When LCI is followed by magnified BLI, it confidently identifies EGC in an MR post-successful HP eradication, outperforming WLI in clinical practice [29].

Further research is essential to assess the effectiveness of LCI in the screening of gastric cancer among the general populace, particularly emphasizing the need for studies centered around EGC. Recent research conducted by Khurelbaatar et al. revealed that LCI, when compared to conventional WLI, notably improves the visibility of early gastric cancer (EGC), regardless of variations in lesion morphology, histology, location, depth of invasion, and HP status. This observation could potentially lead to the reported enhancements in detection rates and reductions in miss rates [30]. In contrast to BLI, LCI exhibits enhanced visibility of EGC, irrespective of the endoscopist's experience [31].

3.1.3 Kyoto classification

The Kyoto classification system for gastritis was formulated primarily to highlight the endoscopic characteristics linked with HP-related gastritis. This system is instrumental in the precise diagnosis of HP infections and in pinpointing the risk factors for gastric carcinoma. In the process of gastroduodenoscopy, it's advised to assess various factors, including nodularity, mucosal atrophy, intestinal metaplasia, enlarged folds, and widespread redness (**Figure 1G–P**). The cumulative score of these elements is used as an index to gauge the risk of gastric cancer. According to this classification, a score of 0 suggests gastritis that is not associated with HP, whereas a score of 2 or higher is indicative of HP-induced gastritis, with a reported diagnostic accuracy of 90% [32].

Notably, LCI has demonstrated utility in evaluating gastritis based on the Kyoto classification [33]. LCI excels in diagnosing mucosal atrophy, intestinal metaplasia, diffuse redness, RAC, spotty redness, and MR from a distant view compared to WLI. Utilizing LCI significantly enhances the detectability of gastroscopic observations in line with the Kyoto Gastritis Classification, presenting a marked improvement over WLI [34]. Moreover, the diagnostic value of the LCI combined score surpasses that of the WLI combined score and each observation index of WLI. These findings suggest that LCI may offer distinct advantages in diagnosing the Kyoto classification of gastritis compared to other IEEs, emphasizing the need for prospective assessments to further validate these potential benefits.

3.1.4 Targeted biopsies

Numerous clinical studies have emphasized the potential of IEEs in identifying mucosal changes, enabling precisely targeted biopsies [11]. In individuals never infected with HP, it was observed that LCI exhibited a greater color difference at the fundic and pyloric mucosal borders compared to WLI. The enhanced detection of atrophic borders with LCI makes it a recommended choice for trans-nasal endoscopy in health check-ups, particularly for identifying individuals at a high risk of gastric carcinoma [5].

4. Mechanism

LCI emerges as an innovative technique in IEEs, utilizing a combination of short-wavelength narrow-band and white-light laser illumination in tandem with traditional WLI. This integration of dual-light modalities enables LCI to gather detailed insights into mucosal surface textures and vascular patterns [35]. In comparison to white light imaging, LCI employs advanced post-processing steps to enhance subtle differences in color tone, with a higher emission intensity of 410 nm influencing the mucosal color of various lesions [34]. Functioning as a cutting-edge IEE technology, LCI excels at highlighting even the slightest differences in mucosal color, making it a powerful tool for the endoscopic diagnosis of gastrointestinal inflammation [1]. The capability of LCI to enhance color differences is particularly beneficial in scenarios of active mucosal inflammation, where hyperemia manifests as noticeable redness. Conversely, mild or inactive inflammation may not exhibit obvious signs during traditional endoscopic examination. LCI, being highly sensitive to color changes, emerges as a convenient and effective tool for detecting these nuanced differences and facilitating a more accurate and differential diagnosis [18].

LCI's unique characteristic of heightened sensitivity to color differences is employed to vividly depict mucosal surface blood vessels and illustrate distinctions in mucosal surface tissue structure, including surface blood vessels [11]. The ELUXEO system was developed with a specific focus on precisely regulating the emission intensity ratio of LED illumination across four colors: blue-violet, blue, green, and red. This setup enables the generation of both white light and short-wavelength narrow-band light. The objective behind this design is to generate high-quality images akin to those produced by LASEREO. With LED-LCI, it is anticipated to achieve diagnostic performance comparable to conventional laser-induced LCI [1].

The enhanced brightness of LCI images is anticipated to increase their utility in detecting subtle irregularities on the gastric surface in patients. Significantly, it has been observed that the orderly pattern of collecting venules, mainly notable in the lesser curvature area, is linked with gastric mucosa not affected by HP and a decreased likelihood of developing gastric cancer [12]. Bright LCI, by highlighting slight irregularities in the surface epithelium even from middle to distant views, significantly improves the ability to detect EGC post-eradication [32]. LCI exhibited the most significant odds ratio compared to factors like elevated morphology and submucosal invasion. Several studies have highlighted the substantial color contrast observed between EGCs and the adjacent mucosa when utilizing LCI. This underscores the crucial role of high color contrast in improving the detectability of EGCs [16, 18].

Fine-tuning color enhancement settings prove instrumental in enhancing the visibility of malignant lesions within the stomach, fostering a clearer color contrast between these lesions and the surrounding mucosa. It is significant to observe that the average scores for visibility, when enhanced with C2 for LCI, were markedly superior in comparison to the results obtained with C1 enhancement [30]. However, it's worth noting that this enhancement, to some extent, compromises the consistency between examiners. To enhance diagnostic accuracy and align with clinical requirements for consistency between examiners, it becomes imperative to improve the consistency of individual observation indices and minimize subjectivity in the evaluation process [36]. Striking the right balance in color enhancement settings is pivotal, ensuring optimal visibility without sacrificing reliability and agreement among different examiners.

5. Artificial intelligence

The integration of artificial intelligence (AI) technology with IEEs is emerging as a potent and innovative diagnostic approach in the evolving landscape of medical imaging. In a pioneering research effort by Sun et al. in China, MATLAB software was applied for the analysis of endoscopic imagery in the LCI mode, specifically targeting the antral region. This research emphasized the extraction and utilization of specific data pertaining to brightness and hue, applying these metrics to the identification and diagnosis of a range of gastric ailments. These include HP infections, gastric atrophy, intestinal metaplasia, and the early stages of gastric cancer [11]. The incorporation of AI, notably through convolutional neural network-based computer-aided diagnosis (CAD) systems, has made significant advancements in gastrointestinal endoscopy. This technology is becoming more widely available and utilized for the detection of HP infection status and gastric cancer [37].

Numerous studies highlight the remarkable capabilities of CAD when integrated with LCI or BLI-bright in discerning the HP infection status [38]. In the study, Nakashima and colleagues demonstrated the effective diagnostic performance of LCI-CAD in categorizing the status of HP infection, effectively differentiating among cases where HP was present, absent, or had been successfully eradicated [39]. The application of AI in diagnostic imaging is expected to alleviate the burden of double-checking, effectively identifying patients in need of follow-up endoscopy while providing crucial support for non-expert endoscopists [40]. In comparison to experienced endoscopists, the study's results revealed that AI exhibits greater sensitivity in diagnosing HP infection, boasting a sensitivity and specificity of 81.9/83.4% and 79/83.2%, respectively. The integration of AI in HP infection diagnosis aims to mitigate interobserver disagreement and reduce time consumption in the diagnostic process. The evolving landscape of AI in conjunction with IEE holds immense promise for advancing the accuracy, efficiency, and accessibility of gastrointestinal diagnostics.

Owing to its elevated rate of HP infections and the extensive need for gastric carcinoma screenings, Japan has emerged as a leading nation in conducting research into the integration of AI within the realm of endoscopic techniques [41]. A prospective pilot study conducted in Japan compared AI-assisted BLI with bright light (AI-BLI-bright), LCI, and WLI in diagnosing HP infection. The performance metrics, specifically the AUC, for both AI-BLI-bright and AI-LCI were impressively elevated, registering at 0.96 and 0.95, respectively. In contrast, AI-WLI demonstrated a lower efficacy with an AUC score of 0.66 [42].

The challenge in the endoscopic diagnosis of HP infection lies in the lack of objective indicators, leading to variations in diagnostic abilities among doctors. Consequently, it becomes crucial to develop methods with universal interpretability, like CAD systems, for the endoscopic assessment of HP infection. The goals of a recent study were to (i) develop an interpretable automated diagnostic system utilizing a support vector machine (SVM) for detecting HP infection, (ii) assess and contrast the diagnostic performance of the AI system with that of endoscopists. The findings indicated that the artificial intelligence system attained levels of accuracy, sensitivity, and specificity, as well as positive and negative predictive values, which were recorded at 87.6%, 90.4%, 85.7%, 80.9%, and 93.1%, respectively. This signifies that the AI system can diagnose HP infection with significant accuracy [39]. The integration of AI systems in endoscopic practices holds great promise for enhancing diagnostic capabilities, standardizing assessments, and contributing to more effective and efficient medical care.

Numerous studies have delved into the CAD of HP infection through deep learning (DL) algorithms. The computer-aided diagnosis system, developed using the GoogLeNet architecture of convolutional neural networks, has shown remarkable efficiency in diagnosing HP infections, thereby illustrating the significant capabilities of deep learning algorithms in the field of gastroenterology [43]. Another CAD, also based on DL algorithms, exhibited significantly higher accuracy and shorter diagnostic times compared to endoscopists in diagnosing HP infection [44].

Concurrently, CAD using IEE images has been actively explored. A computer-aided diagnosis system, powered by deep learning algorithms, demonstrated significantly enhanced precision in detecting anomalies using BLI-bright and LCI, in contrast to the results obtained with traditional WLI [45]. Similarly, a CAD system based on a conventional support vector machine, utilizing LCI, demonstrated diagnostic yields on part with those of expert endoscopists [39].

In broadening its application, CAD encompasses the use of the Kyoto criteria for gastritis in the endoscopic identification of HP infections. A predictive model, employing a machine learning approach and incorporating endoscopic features derived from the Kyoto classification of gastritis, demonstrated a high level of diagnostic accuracy for determining HP infection status. This accuracy was found to be comparable to evaluations made by experienced endoscopists [43]. These findings underscore the growing potential of CAD, both with DL algorithms and traditional methods, in revolutionizing the accuracy, efficiency, and objectivity of diagnosing HP infection and related gastric conditions.

6. Education

Fukuda et al. brought attention to a noteworthy challenge in lesion recognition, reporting that malignant lesions appearing redder than the surrounding mucosa on WLI may manifest as purple on LCI. This color shift could potentially lead to the oversight of malignant lesions, even in the presence of surface irregularities. Therefore, it has become imperative to enhance educational efforts to heighten recognition of the importance attached to the purple hue observed in LCI [46]. Despite the complexities involved, assessing HP infection via indicators such as widespread erythema, loss of the typical collecting venule pattern, and mucus adhesion when using LCI proves to be a dependable method. These indicators are deemed attainable skills for gastrointestinal endoscopists, covering a range of expertise from novices to seasoned professionals. Nonetheless, it is underscored that additional research, particularly with a focus on practitioners of varying experience levels, is crucial to fully comprehending the benefits of LCI in the educational spectrum of endoscopy. Analyzing results before and after systematic training will contribute to a comprehensive assessment of LCI's efficacy [18].

In an extensive research project, clarity levels and interclass correlation coefficients (ICCs) were utilized to evaluate the visibility and consistency among different raters for both LCI and BLI-bright, relative to traditional WLI. This assessment was conducted based on the findings observed through endoscopy, which were in line with the criteria outlined in the Kyoto Classification of Gastritis. Notably, statistically significant differences in visibility scores for LCI were observed between trainees and experts, particularly in categories such as spotty, patchy, and MR. Trainees exhibited significantly higher visibility scores than experts for spotty redness observed through LCI, suggesting that LCI may enhance diagnostic performance in the assessment of spotty redness by non-experts [10].

Building on this insight, our team embarked on an initiative to integrate LCI with the Kyoto Classification of Gastritis, forming a training model tailored for general practitioners (GPs). Expert endoscopists' analysis of the Kyoto Classification of Gastritis revealed that gastroscopic mucosal manifestations such as mucosal atrophy, hematin deposition, mucosal swelling, and the presence of sticky mucus influenced their assessment of HP infection. Subsequent to the training program, there was a notable enhancement in the overall scores achieved by GPs in the questionnaire. Additionally, the time taken to complete the questionnaire was comparable between the GPs and established gastroenterology specialists. Following training, general practitioners' questionnaire scores improved based on images observed in both WLI and LCI modes. Notably, the score achieved with the LCI mode was superior to that obtained with the WLI mode. The conclusion of the study is that the Kyoto Classification of Gastritis combined with LCI improves the ability of GPs to diagnose HP infection through endoscopic images.

7. Conclusion

LCI observation mode can enhance the diagnosis rate of HP infection-related gastritis, providing accurate diagnostic performance and precise localization. LCI demonstrates a high level of diagnostic accuracy in identifying HP infections, including their precise locations, when contrasted with traditional white-light endoscopic methods. Additionally, LCI shows promise in enhancing the precision of sample collection for HP culture and its antibiotic sensitivity analysis. Integrating LCI with the Kyoto Classification of Gastritis could potentially elevate the effectiveness of diagnosing HP infections or confirming their eradication during endoscopic procedures. This advancement might significantly bolster the capabilities of gastrointestinal endoscopists and general practitioners in diagnosing HP infections through endoscopic imaging.

Acknowledgements

This study was supported by the Guangdong Basic and Applied Basic Research Foundation (2022B1515130004). Thanks to Lanfeng Xue, Yujia Guo, and Haiyun Zhuang who performed the experiments and meta-analysis, as well as the figures collection.

Conflict of interest

The authors declare no conflict of interest.

Author details

Yu Chen[1*] and Weiguang Qiao[2]

1 Department of Gastroenterology, The Seventh Affiliated Hospital of Southern Medical University, Guangdong, China

2 Department of Gastroenterology, Nanfang Hospital, Southern Medical University, Guangdong, China

*Address all correspondence to: askasky@126.com

References

[1] Osawa H, Miura Y, Takezawa T, et al. Linked color imaging and blue laser imaging for gastrointestinal screening. Clinical Endoscopy. 2018;**51**:513-526. DOI: 10.5946/ce.2018.132

[2] Kanzaki H, Takenaka R, Kawahara Y, Kawai D, Obayashi Y, Baba Y, et al. Linked color imaging (LCI), a novel image-enhanced endoscopy technology, emphasizes the color of early gastric cancer. Endoscopy International Open. 2017;**5**:E1005-E1013. DOI: 10.1055/s-0043-117881

[3] Fukuda H, Miura Y, Hayashi Y, et al. Linked color imaging technology facilitates the early detection of fat gastric cancers. Clinical Journal of Gastroenterology. 2015;**8**:385-389. DOI: 10.1007/s12328-015-0612-9

[4] Yashima K, Onoyama T, Kurumi H, et al. Current status and future perspective of linked color imaging for gastric cancer screening: A literature review. Journal of Gastroenterology. Jan 2023;**58**(1):1-13. DOI: 10.1007/s00535-022-01934-z. Epub 2022 Oct 26. Erratum in: J Gastroenterol. 2023 May;58(5):514. PMID: 36287268; PMCID: PMC9825522

[5] Chatrangsun B, Vilaichone RK. Endoscopic diagnosis for *H. pylori* infection: White light imaging (WLI) vs. image-enhanced endoscopy (IEE). Asian Pacific Journal of Cancer Prevention. 2021;**22**(9):3031-3038. DOI: 10.31557/APJCP.2021.22.9.3031

[6] Malfertheiner P, Megraud F, O'Morain C, et al. Current concepts in the management of *Helicobacter pylori* infection: The Maastricht III Consensus Report. Gut. 2007;**56**:772-781. DOI: 10.1136/gut.2006.101634

[7] Uemura N, Okamoto S, Yamamoto S, et al. *Helicobacter pylori* infection and the development of gastric cancer. The New England Journal of Medicine. 2001;**345**:784-789. DOI: 10.1056/NEJMoa001999

[8] Dohi O, Yagi N, Onozawa Y, et al. Linked color imaging improves endoscopic diagnosis of active *Helicobacter pylori* infection. Endoscopy International Open. 2016;**4**:E800-E805. DOI: 10.1055/s-0042-109049

[9] Hiraoka Y, Miura Y, Osawa H, et al. Linked color imaging demonstrates characteristic findings in semi-pedunculated gastric adenocarcinoma in *Helicobacter pylori*-negative normal mucosa. Clinical Endoscopy. Jan 2021;**54**(1):136-138. DOI: 10.5946/ce.2020.059

[10] Wang L, Lin XC, Li HL, Yang XS, Zhang L, Li X, et al. Clinical significance and influencing factors of linked color imaging technique in real-time diagnosis of active *Helicobacter pylori* infection. Chinese Medical Journal. 2019;**132**(20):2395-2401. DOI: 10.1097/CM9.0000000000000486

[11] Xiu JZ, Bing N, Juan NJ, Yu HP. Comparison between the linked color and white light imaging combined score in the evaluation of high-risk population of gastric cancer. The Turkish Journal of Gastroenterology. 2021;**32**(10):859-869. DOI: 10.5152/tjg.2021.20799

[12] Ishida T, Dohi O, Yoshida N, et al. Enhanced visibility in evaluating gastric cancer 1 and *Helicobacter pylori*-associated gastritis using linked color imaging with a light-emitting diode light source. Digestive Diseases and Sciences. 2022;**67**:2367-2371. DOI: 10.1007/s10620-021-07234-5

[13] Chen TH, Hsu CM, Cheng HT, et al. Linked color imaging can help gastric *Helicobacter pylori* infection diagnosis during endoscopy. Journal of the Chinese Medical Association. 2018;**81**:1033-1037. DOI: 10.1016/j.jcma.2018.03.006

[14] Iwamuro M, Sakae H, Kanzaki H, Okada H. Diffuse redness in linked color imaging is useful for diagnosing current *Helicobacter pylori* infection in the stomach. Journal of General and Family Medicine. 2018;**19**(5):176-177. DOI: 10.1002/jgf2.195 PMID: 30186732

[15] Majima A, Dohi O, Takayama S, et al. Linked color imaging identifies important risk factors associated with gastric cancer after the successful eradication of *Helicobacter pylori*. Gastrointestinal Endoscopy. 2019;**90**:763-769. DOI: 10.1016/j.gie.2019.06.043

[16] Kitagawa Y, Suzuki T, Nankinzan R, Ishigaki A, Furukawa K, Sugita O, et al. Comparison of endoscopic visibility and miss rate for early gastric cancers after *Helicobacter pylori* eradication with white-light imaging versus linked color imaging. Digestive Endoscopy. 2020;**32**(5):769-777. DOI: 10.1111/den.13585

[17] Nishikawa Y, Ikeda Y, Murakami H, Hori SI, Hino K, Sasaki C, et al. Classification of atrophic mucosal patterns on blue Laser imaging for endoscopic diagnosis of *Helicobacter pylori*-related gastritis: A retrospective, observational study. PLoS ONE. 2018;**13**:e0193197. DOI: 10.1371/journal.pone.0193197

[18] Fukuda H, Miura Y, Osawa H, et al. Linked color imaging can enhance the recognition of early gastric cancer by high color contrast with the surrounding gastric intestinal metaplasia. Journal of Gastroenterology. 2019;**54**:396-406. DOI: 10.1007/s00535-018-1515-6

[19] Ono S, Dohi O, Yagi N, et al. Accuracies of endoscopic diagnosis of *Helicobacter pylori*-gastritis: A multicenter prospective study using white light imaging and linked color imaging. Digestion. 2020;**101**:624-630. DOI: 10.1159/000501634

[20] Shu X, Wu G, Zhang Y, et al. Diagnostic value of linked color imaging based on endoscopy for gastric intestinal metaplasia: A systematic review and meta-analysis. Annals of Translational Medicine. 2021;**9**:506. DOI: 10.21037/atm-21-1051

[21] Mizukami K, Ogawa R, Okamoto K, et al. Objective endoscopic analysis with linked color imaging for gastric mucosal atrophy: A pilot study. Gastroenterology Research and Practice. 2017;**2017**:5054237. DOI: 10.1155/2017/5054237

[22] Esaki M, Minoda Y, Ihara E. In living color: Linked color imaging for the detection of early gastric cancer. Digestive Diseases and Sciences. 2022;**67**:1922-1924. DOI: 10.1007/s10620-021-07235-4

[23] Kyung Yoo I, Lee H, Il Kim Y, Young Cho J, Sik LW. Clinical usefulness of linked color imaging for detection and characterization of undifferentiated type early gastric cancer. The Turkish Journal of Gastroenterology. 2023;**34**(4):356-363. DOI: 10.5152/tjg.2023.22684

[24] Jiang ZX, Nong B, Liang LX, Yan YD, Zhang G. Differential diagnosis of *Helicobacter pylori*-associated gastritis with the linked-color imaging score. Digestive and Liver Disease 2019;**51**(12):1665-1670. DOI: 10.1016/j.dld.2019.06.024

[25] Hatta W, Gotoda T, Oyama T, et al. A scoring system to stratify curability after endoscopic submucosal dissection for early gastric cancer: "eCura system". The American Journal of Gastroenterology. 2017;**112**:874-881. DOI: 10.1038/ajg.2017.95

[26] Lee SP, Lee J, Kae SH, Jang HJ, Koh DH, Jung JH, et al. The role of linked color imaging in endoscopic diagnosis of *Helicobacter pylori* associated gastritis. Scandinavian Journal of Gastroenterology. 2020;**55**(9):1114-1120. DOI: 10.1080/00365521.2020.1794025

[27] Muto M, Yao K, Kaise M, et al. Magnifying endoscopy simple diagnostic algorithm for early gastric cancer (MESDA-G). Digestive Endoscopy. 2016;**28**:379-393. DOI: 10.1111/den.12638

[28] Ono S, Abiko S, Kato M. Linked color imaging enhances gastric cancer in gastric intestinal metaplasia. Digestive Endoscopy. 2017;**29**(2):230-231. DOI: 10.1111/den.12757

[29] Dohi O, Ishida T, Yoshida N. Linked color imaging followed by magnifying blue laser imaging identifies early gastric cancer in map-like redness after successful *Helicobacter pylori* eradication. Digestive Endoscopy. 2020;**32**(5):e109-e111. DOI: 10.1111/den.13708

[30] Khurelbaatar T, Miura Y, Osawa H, et al. Usefulness of linked color imaging for the detection of obscure early gastric cancer: Multivariate analysis of 508 lesions. Digestive Endoscopy. 2022;**34**:1012-1020. DOI: 10.1111/den.14221

[31] Matsumura S, Dohi O, Yamada N, et al. Improved visibility of early gastric cancer after successful *Helicobacter pylori* eradication with image-enhanced endoscopy: A multi-institutional study using video clips. Journal of Clinical Medicine. 2021;**10**:3649

[32] Dohi O, Majima A, Naito Y, Yoshida T, Ishida T, Azuma Y, et al. Can image-enhanced endoscopy improve the diagnosis of Kyoto classification of gastritis in the clinical setting? Digestive Endoscopy. 2020;**32**(2):191-203. DOI: 10.1111/den.13540

[33] Toyoshima O, Nishizawa T, Koike K. Endoscopic Kyoto classification of *Helicobacter pylori* infection and gastric cancer risk diagnosis. World Journal of Gastroenterology. 2020;**26**:466-477. DOI: 10.3748/wjg.v26.i5.466

[34] Takeda T, Asaoka D, Nojiri S, et al. Linked color imaging and Kyoto classification of gastritis: Evaluation of visibility and inter-rater reliability. Digestion. 2020;**101**:598-607. DOI: 10.1159/000501534

[35] Kawai Y, Sugimoto M, Hamada M, Iwata E, Niikura R, Nagata N, et al. Linked color imaging effectively detects the endoscopic atrophic border in transnasal endoscopy. Journal of Clinical Biochemistry and Nutrition. 2022;**70**(3):290-296. DOI: 10.3164/jcbn.21-145

[36] Hiraoka Y, Miura Y, Osawa H, Nomoto Y, Takahashi H, Tsunoda M, et al. Appropriate color enhancement settings for blue laser imaging facilitates the diagnosis of early gastric cancer with high color contrast. Journal of Gastric Cancer. 2021;**21**(2):142-154. DOI: 10.5230/jgc.2021.21.e13 Epub 2021 Jun 17

[37] Sun X, Bi Y, Dong T, Min M, Shen W, Xu Y, et al. Linked color imaging benefits the endoscopic diagnosis of distal gastric diseases. Scientific Reports. 2017;7:5638. DOI: 10.1038/s41598-017-05847-3

[38] Kanesaka T, Lee TC, Uedo N, Lin KP, et al. Computer-aided diagnosis for identifying and delineating early gastric cancers in magnifying narrow-band imaging. Gastrointestinal Endoscopy. May 2018;**87**(5):1339-1344. DOI: 10.1016/j.gie.2017.11.029

[39] Nakashima H, Kawahira H, Kawachi H, et al. Artificial intelligence diagnosis of *Helicobacter pylori* infection using blue laser imaging-bright and linked color imaging: A singlecenter prospective study. Annals of Gastroenterology. 2018;**31**:462-468. DOI: 10.20524/aog.2018.0269

[40] Nakashima H, Kawahira H, Kawachi H, et al. Endoscopic threecategorical diagnosis of *Helicobacter pylori* infection using linked color imaging and deep learning: A single-center prospective study (with video). Gastric Cancer. 2020;**23**:1033-1040. DOI: 10.1007/s10120-020-01077-1

[41] Abe S, Oda I. How can endoscopists adapt and collaborate with artificial intelligence for early gastric cancer detection? Digestive Endoscopy. 2021;**33**:98-99. DOI: 10.1111/den.13751

[42] Bang CS, Lee JJ, Baik GH. Artificial intelligence for the prediction of *Helicobacter pylori* infection in endoscopic images: Systematic review and meta-analysis of diagnostic test accuracy. Journal of Medical Internet Research. 2020;**22**:e21983. DOI: 10.2196/21983

[43] Yasuda T, Hiroyasu T, Hiwa S, Okada Y, Hayashi S, Nakahata Y, et al. Potential of automatic diagnosis system with linked color imaging for diagnosis of *Helicobacter pylori* infection. Digestive Endoscopy. 2020;**32**(3):373-381. DOI: 10.1111/den.13509

[44] Itoh T, Kawahira H, Nakashima H, et al. Deep learning analyzes *Helicobacter pylori* infection by upper gastrointestinal endoscopy images. Endoscopy International Open. 2018;**6**:E139-E144. DOI: 10.1055/s-0043-120830

[45] Shichijo S, Nomura S, Aoyama K, et al. Application of convolutional neural networks in the diagnosis of *Helicobacter pylori* infection based on endoscopic images. EBioMedicine. 2017;**25**:106-111. DOI: 10.1016/j.ebiom.2017.10.014

[46] Yoshii S, Mabe K, Watano K, et al. Validity of endoscopic features for the diagnosis of *Helicobacter pylori* infection status based on the Kyoto classification of gastritis. Digestive Endoscopy. Jan 2020;**32**(1):74-83. DOI: 10.1111/den.13486

Section 2

Treatment of *Helicobacter pylori* Infection

Chapter 5

Antibiotic Resistance, Susceptibility Testing and Stewardship in *Helicobacter pylori* Infection

Lok Ka Lam and Ka Shing Cheung

Abstract

It is promising to observe a worldwide decrease in the prevalence of *Helicobacter pylori* (*H. pylori*), yet consistent efforts are required to enhance treatment regimens in accordance with antibiotic stewardship in the era of growing antibiotic resistance. Various molecular mechanisms are responsible for antibiotic resistance, and thanks to technological advancements, our understanding of these mechanisms has improved, which facilitated the assessment of antibiotic susceptibility to *H. pylori*. Progress made in next-generation sequencing technology could potentially herald a new era, encouraging the routine use of non-invasive tests to gather data on antibiotic resistance. It is crucial that studies and clinical guidelines ensure the proposed treatment can consistently meet an acceptable level of eradication rate, taking into account the variations in antibiotic resistance across different populations. Future investigations should strive to refine the duration and dosage and reduce side effects of treatment regimens. Through personalized medicine, better treatment strategies can be formulated. It is equally important to actively encourage patient adherence to these treatments through all available strategies. Collaboration among local, regional, and international bodies is necessary to reinforce antibiotic stewardship in *H. pylori* treatment.

Keywords: *H. pylori*, vonoprazan, stewardship, NGS, WGS

1. Introduction

Helicobacter pylori (*H. pylori)* is a Gram-negative bacterium that preferentially colonizes the antrum, but may infect any part of the stomach to cause gastritis. Although most patients infected with *H. pylori* are asymptomatic, approximately 10–15% develop peptic ulcer disease [1], and 1–3% develop stomach cancer and lymphoma [2, 3]. The carcinogenic evolution of *H. pylori-induced* chronic gastritis follows the Correa's cascade [4] via a stepwise process from active gastritis, to precursor lesions of gastric cancer, and finally adenocarcinoma. Gastric cancer is the fifth most common cancer and the fourth leading cause of cancer-related mortality across the globe [5].

H. pylori infection usually lasts for life unless it is treated. The recognition of *H. pylori* as an infectious disease and its associated complications by the Kyoto consensus [6] and Maastricht/Florence Consensus [7], has led to a unanimous agreement on the necessity of treating all individuals diagnosed with *H. pylori* infection, irrespective of symptoms. Successful eradication of *H. pylori* aids not only in peptic ulcer healing [8, 9] but also plays an important role in the prevention of gastric cancer both primarily and secondarily [10], thus significantly reducing the incidence and mortality of gastric cancer [11–13].

Eradication of *H. pylori* requires a combination of gastric acid suppressants and antibiotics. Various treatment regimens have been adopted based on local antibiotic resistance patterns, drug availability, and patient acceptability. Standard triple therapy consisting of amoxicillin or metronidazole, clarithromycin, and a proton pump inhibitor (PPI) was the gold standard in the treatment of *H. pylori* infections during the 90s [14, 15]. Given the emergence of clarithromycin resistance, a substantial decline in its efficacy to levels below 80–85% has been observed [16, 17]. Bismuth-based quadruple therapy consisting of bismuth, PPI, metronidazole, and tetracycline, has been shown to achieve over 90% success rate [18, 19] and has been increasingly recommended as first-line treatment [7, 20, 21]. Resistance in metronidazole varies among different regions, with a resistance rate of 43.6% across the US [22] and 78% in China [23]. Increasing the metronidazole dose and duration may overcome antibiotic resistance [24]. While sequential regimen is discouraged [25], the marginal effect of metronidazole resistance in affecting therapeutic outcome allows quadruple therapy to remain as an effective eradication regimen [26].

Antibiotic stewardship, encompassing the judicious use of antibiotics, selecting optimal treatment regimens (including the appropriate antibiotics, dosing, and duration of treatment), and ensuring sustainable access to antibiotics, is increasingly advocated to put forward better clinical outcomes for patients and minimize subsequent resistance [27]. In order to provide information for designing optimal treatment regimens, routine susceptibility testing has been recommended to be performed even before first-line treatment in compliance with antibiotic stewardship [14, 15]. Recently, antibiotic susceptibility testing obtained via culture or molecular testing for *H. pylori* eradication has been more readily available [7, 20, 21]. This shifts the paradigm toward personalized medicine in which *H. pylori* treatment regimens can be tailored according to local resistance patterns and individual profiles.

This review will provide an overview of the current resistance patterns and mechanisms of *H. pylori* antibiotics, as well as different antibiotic susceptibility testing methods. We will emphasize the importance of antibiotic stewardship, and illustrate how susceptibility testing has become an integral part of this paradigm. We will also highlight the new direction of *H. pylori* eradication and the emergence of potential therapeutic options.

2. Antibiotic resistance in *Helicobacter pylori*

H. pylori treatment is challenged by high and continuously rising antibiotic resistance. There are two types of resistance—primary and secondary. Primary antibiotic resistance is identified in patients who are naïve to *H. pylori* eradication treatment, whereas secondary or acquired resistance emerges following one or more failed attempts at eradication [28]. Eradication of *H. pylori* infection now relies heavily on local antibiotic resistance patterns and patients' prior antibiotic exposure.

A meta-analysis by Savoldi et al. in 2018 has reported a pooled prevalence of >15% in both primary and secondary resistance of *H. pylori* to key antibiotics (clarithromycin, metronidazole, and levofloxacin) in most World Health Organization (WHO) regions [28], which exceed the common threshold for choosing alternative empiric *H. pylori* eradication treatment [7, 21]. Resistance profile differs among regions. In the Asia-Pacific region, a meta-analysis found an overall prevalence of primary antibiotic resistance of *H. pylori* to clarithromycin, metronidazole, and levofloxacin between 1990 and 2022 to be 22%, 52%, and 25%, respectively [29]. Prevalence varied considerably across study periods. From 1990–2000 to 2016–2022, the prevalence increased from 7% to 30% for clarithromycin, 37% to 61% for metronidazole, and 9% to 35% for levofloxacin, but remained consistently low for both amoxicillin and tetracycline at less than 6% [29]. In the United States, the pooled resistance prevalence of clarithromycin, levofloxacin, and metronidazole from 2011 to 2021 was 31.5%, 37.6%, and 42.1%, respectively [30]. Similar trends have also been observed in Africa and Latin America [31, 32]. Conversely, primary resistance to key antibiotics showed a decreasing trend in Europe. From 2013–2016 to 2017–2020, the primary resistance of clarithromycin, metronidazole, and levofloxacin decreased from 25% to 20%, 33% to 24.5%, and 20.5% to 18%, respectively [33].

The resistance mechanisms that *H. pylori* evolved are multifarious. The exact nature of such genetic modifications varies depending on the specific class of antibiotics involved. Most often, it is due to chromosomally encoded mutations [34–36]. Clarithromycin resistance is frequently caused by 23S rRNA gene mutation [37–40], while levofloxacin resistance is commonly due to *gyrA* mutations [37, 41]. For metronidazole resistance, the mutational changes display greater diversity, and the genotype-phenotype correlation is more complex [37]. Mutations in *RdxA* and *FrxA* gene, which encodes NADPH nitroreductase, are most frequently reported [42]. Levofloxacin resistance is primarily attributed to point mutations within the quinolones resistance-determining region (QRDR) of the *gyrA* gene, or, less often, the *gyrB* gene [43]. Amoxicillin resistance is mainly attributed to mutations in the penicillin-binding proteins (PBP), namely PBP1, PBP2, and PBP3 [44]. Beyond these genetic adaptations, *H. pylori* can also resist antibiotics through physiological defenses such as efflux pumps and biofilm formation, which can further complicate treatment [45].

Multidrug resistance (MDR) is defined as non-susceptibility to three or more antibiotics of different classes. The prevalence of MDR is characterized by a regional variation and appears to be changing over time. A significant concern is the concurrent resistance to both clarithromycin and metronidazole, with prevalence of approximately 8–15% in Europe [28, 33, 46], 6–11% in Asia [28], and 3–11% in the Americas [22, 28, 30]. In China, double, triple, quadruple, and quintuple resistance rates were reported to be 23, 20, 6, and 4%, respectively between 1998 and 2007 [47]. A study in the Tibet Autonomous Region of China has further demonstrated a high resistance rate where only 3 (2.0%) out of the 153 *H. pylori* strains isolated were susceptible to all the seven tested antibiotics [48]. In Spain, triple resistance decreased from 3.3% in 2013 to 1.8% in 2015, and then increased to 2.4% in 2017 [49]. The exact mechanism of MDR is not well known, but various mutations that simultaneously induce resistance to different classes of antibiotics are believed to confer a cumulative MDR profile. Apart from biofilm formation and increased efflux pump commonly described in single drug resistance, additional mechanisms include coccoid formation. The coccoid form is an inactive form of *H. pylori* that slows metabolism to facilitate survival [50], which substantially increases the minimum inhibitory concentrations (MIC) of different antibiotics. Subsequent ultrastructural modifications in the cell membrane and metabolic pathways contribute to the development of MDR by reducing drug target exposure and drug penetration [51].

Heteroresistance is a term indicating the diverse responses to specific antibiotics by bacterial subpopulations in the same patient, which do not respond to antibiotic therapy *in vitro* or *in vivo* [52]. Currently, there are no recommendations for the treatment of *H. pylori* infections caused by heteroresistant strains in the clinical setting. Given the great interest in developing new strategies to enhance the eradication rate of *H. pylori* eradication therapy, apart from strategies tackling the single- or multi-drug resistance, future guidelines should include a personalized aspect in the protocol to address heteroresistance to *H. pylori*.

3. Antimicrobial susceptibility testing for *Helicobacter pylori*

H. pylori treatment regimen is considered to be acceptable if it achieves at least 90% cure rate [17], while an optimized regimen should reliably achieve ≥95% cure rates [53]. *H. pylori's* resistance to key antibiotics like clarithromycin, levofloxacin, or metronidazole is very common. The increasing resistance of *H. pylori* to antibiotic therapy necessitates local availability of susceptibility tests for individuals, as well as regional and national monitoring programs, to develop eradication strategies. Antimicrobial susceptibility testing (AST) for *H. pylori* can be primarily categorized into two types: culture-based techniques and molecular-based methods. The details of each approach, including their application, performance, advantages, and disadvantages, will be discussed below.

3.1 Culture-based techniques

Culture-based techniques are considered the gold standard for AST of *H. pylori*. These techniques employ the phenotypic identification of susceptibility and resistance based on the minimal inhibitory concentration (MIC) of the tested antibiotic [54, 55]. Traditional culture-based techniques can be categorized into quantitative or qualitative methods. Qualitative methods, for instance, the disc diffusion method, allow broad categorization of antibiotic susceptibility or resistance without an exact MIC value. Quantitative methods include agar dilution, gradient diffusion susceptibility testing (also known as the E-test), and broth dilution method, which express results numerically. Details of each method are outlined below.

3.1.1 Disk diffusion method

In the disc diffusion test, filter paper discs impregnated with various pre-defined concentrations of antibiotics are placed on an agar plate that has been pre-swabbed uniformly with pure bacterial culture. The agar plate is then incubated at a certain temperature optimal for the growth of a microorganism. The incubation time is dependent on the natural growth rate of the tested microorganism. During the incubation, the antibiotic diffuses from the disk to the agar, with the concentration decreasing as the distance to the disk increases. If the microorganism is susceptible to an antibiotic in the disk, there is a clear inhibition zone around the disk. The size of the inhibition zone indicates categorial results, for instance, susceptible, intermediate, and resistant, and can be related to MIC. The disk diffusion method is the simplest and most economical routine susceptibility testing. However, it is generally not recommended for *H. pylori,* a slow-growing bacterium. Disk diffusion has been validated in France to detect macrolide resistance [56]. However, this method has not been validated for the other antibiotics.

3.1.2 Agar dilution method

The agar dilution method, which is considered the reference method to compare other techniques, was first proposed by the Clinical Laboratory Standard Institute (CLSI) as the method to be used for *H. pylori* clarithromycin susceptibility testing, which later extended to testing of other antibiotics such as amoxicillin, rifabutin, ciprofloxacin, etc. Maastricht VI Florence consensus report has affirmed the agar dilution method as the gold standard for AST. Metronidazole, however, is a special case in which inter- and intra-laboratory reproducibility is lacking, and a correlation between the susceptibility results and *H. pylori* eradication is not evident [57]. Therefore, since the Maastricht III 2005 consensus report, routine metronidazole susceptibility testing has been discouraged.

3.1.3 E-test

E-test is a method derived from the disk diffusion test that provides quantitative MIC results. In the E-test, a commercially available thin plastic test strip with a continuous gradient of antibiotic is placed on an agar plate, which has been pre-swabbed uniformly with pure bacterial culture. The agar plate is then incubated during which a continuous gradient of concentrations of antibiotic is created at the intermediate vicinity of the test strip. Since the concentration gradient remains stable for at least 18–24 hours, the long enough duration allows most fastidious and non-fastidious microorganisms, including *H. pylori*, to be tested. After overnight incubation, a clear ellipse-shaped inhibition zone appears along the test strip where the MIC value could be read from the scale point, taken as the intersection between the edge of the ellipse and the strip. The E-test method has the advantage of being a quantitative method with a direct expression of MICs. Except for metronidazole, a good correlation has been found between the E-test and the standard agar dilution method.

3.1.4 Broth dilution method

In the broth dilution test, a known number of microorganisms are inoculated into tubes containing dilution of antibiotics where MIC will be measured. The broth dilution method has the advantage of being adaptable to automation. It is typically used to test pure isolates of non-fastidious aerobic microorganisms, which are easily grown by overnight incubation. However, it is not commonly used for *H. pylori* because of the difficulty in growing this bacterium in broth. Supplementation of media such as brucella broth or Mueller Hinton broth allows a good correlation with the E-test, except for metronidazole.

Susceptibility testing is currently available from a number of diagnostic laboratories. Given the slow-growing nature of *H. pylori*, the broth dilution method is not routinely used as previously mentioned [37, 58, 59]. For routine testing, the minimum is to test a macrolide. The disk diffusion method, with an erythromycin disk, is the simplest cost-effective strategy. To quantify the exact MIC, an E-test or agar dilution method can be used. The agar dilution method has proven reliable and can be adapted for simultaneous testing of multiple *H. pylori* strains [55, 60]. E-test quantifies the disc diffusion method and strongly correlates with the agar dilution method for most antibiotics. The only exception is metronidazole due to the absence of anaerobic preincubation of plates used [58, 59], lack of reproducibility, and low predictive value for treatment efficacy. If necessary, the best method is agar dilution or its simplified version, known as the break-point method. The breakpoint susceptibility test consists of inoculating antibiotic concentration equal to the breakpoint concentration, which defines resistance to classify the strains as susceptible, intermediary, or resistant. Compared to the agar diffusion method for the metronidazole susceptibility test, a correlation of 94% has been shown [61], although reproducibility was not studied.

Culture and susceptibility testing are performed using fresh or frozen gastric biopsies obtained via endoscopy. Adequate tissue sampling and proper handling are needed for accurate antimicrobial analysis. At least 2 biopsies (1 from the corpus and 1 from the antrum) should be taken, preferably using large cup forceps. Samples collected have to be placed in a transport medium (e.g., Brucella broth with 20% glycerol, Portagerm pylori, or an equivalent). Biopsy specimens should be transported and processed for culture as soon as possible, ideally within six hours. If processing is delayed, refrigeration is recommended. Biopsies frozen at −70°C in Brucella broth with glycerol remain stable for months [62].

The efficacy of these methods greatly depends on the conditions under which the tests are performed, and the quality of the samples provided. Factors such as the biopsy site, the number of samples taken, the quality of the sample, the time interval between sampling and culture, and even transport conditions like temperature and air exposure can significantly affect the reliability of these methods [63, 64]. Consequently, the process becomes costly, labor-intensive, and time-consuming, often taking up to two weeks to yield results [37, 63]. *H. pylori* culture, an integral part of this process, is complex due to the bacterium's requirement for a microaerophilic environment and a specialized medium that doesn't interfere with the AST. In specific to metronidazole, redox variations in the medium can affect metronidazole susceptibility testing [35, 64]. Furthermore, the interpretation of results is subjective and highly dependent on experimental conditions [65]. A recent systematic review underscored these limitations by revealing a failure of bacterial growth in about 20% of the cases studied [66]. The study also found that, although culture-tailored treatment achieved an optimal eradication rate of over 90% when used before first- and second-line regimens [7, 53], it was ineffective after two or more eradication failures [66]. To tackle the time, cost, and intensive labor required for culture-based AST methods, molecular (or genotypic AST) is recommended as an alternative for the detection of AST.

3.2 Molecular-based techniques

Molecular-based techniques employ the genotypic detection of resistance to the tested antibiotics. These methods facilitate the identification of specific mutations that lead to antibiotic resistance. Molecular-based tests can be categorized into polymerase chain reaction (PCR) assays and next-generation sequencing (NGS).

3.2.1 PCR-based assay

The PCR assay uses nucleic acid amplification to detect specific genes responsible for antibiotic resistance. The microorganisms isolated from specimen samples are lysed with their DNA extracted and fragmented. Targeted genes subject to antibiotic resistance are identified from genomic analysis of the amplified DNA fragments.

Common PCR-based assays include real-time polymerase chain reaction (RT-PCR), hybridization with oligonucleotide probes, and analysis of restriction fragment length polymorphism (RFLP). RT-PCR is a repetitive cycle of target DNA synthesis that allows the determination of the presence of *H. pylori* and mutation types, as well as its quantification. Fluorescence *in situ* hybridization (FISH) is used to detect *H. pylori* antibiotic resistance via histological preparations, where the result is interpreted under a fluorescent microscope. The PCR-RFLP method is based on the amplification of DNA gene regions and selective cleavage of PCR products using restriction endonucleases that recognize mutation sites.

Most available PCR-based assays primarily focus on testing common point mutations in 23S rRNA for clarithromycin resistance and in *gyrA* for levofloxacin resistance [37, 63, 67]. However, the mechanism of metronidazole resistance is not well understood, and thus, a definitive panel of point mutations accounting for metronidazole resistance has not yet been described [68].

Recent advancements in assays for detecting clarithromycin resistance can be applied to both biopsy and stool specimens, enabling simultaneous detection of the presence of *H. pylori* and clarithromycin resistance. Some assays can even differentiate between high and low resistance levels based on the point mutation [69, 70]. However, the sensitivity of molecular assays in detecting *H. pylori* using stool samples varies—some studies have reported high sensitivity up to 93.8% [71], and others have found lower sensitivity ranging from 63% to 84% compared to gastric biopsy specimens [72–74]. This discrepancy may be explained by variable DNA extraction methods and the molecular assays selected in the testing process. For instance, the use of FFPE gastric biopsy samples may lead to false negatives, as the DNA can be broken into smaller fragments by the fixative [75–77]. The accuracy of these assays can be influenced by factors such as the sample's quality and the condition and purity of the DNA. Lately, quantitative PCR using gastric fluid collected via string-test has been proposed for the detection of *H. pylori* and its resistance against clarithromycin and levofloxacin [78].

Gastric fluid collection via string test was done by asking the patient to swallow and retain a gelatin capsule containing a cotton string absorbed with water for one hour. Compared to conventional culturing techniques, string-qPCR test allows resistance test to be done in a non-invasive, low-cost, simple, and rapid manner [79]. The high eradication rate greater than 90% indicates its feasibility and applicability in clinical practice [80].

3.2.2 Next-generation sequencing

The Sanger sequencing method is the analysis of the nucleotide sequence of the studied DNA section. Instead of requiring two primers from opposite strands, which is required in PCR amplification, Sanger sequencing allows amplification using only one primer. It has the advantage over PCR methods in reducing errors associated with improper DNA amplification and subsequent interpretation. With Sanger sequencing, sequences up to 1000 base pairs long could be read in one cycle with a high accuracy of 98% [81]. The precision and robustness of Sanger sequencing contribute significantly to the scientific basis of clinical investigations. However, the inability to detect large deletions or duplications of the sequence has moved Sanger sequencing (also known as first-generation sequencing) to next-generation sequencing.

Next-generation sequencing (NGS), a step beyond Sanger and Maxam-Gilbert sequencing, is a potential substitute for culture-based methods and current

PCR-based assays. These novel methods enable the identification of complex genetic variants involved in antibiotic resistance, offering an advantage through their ability to perform massively parallel sequencing of DNA and RNA at a relatively lower cost [82]. Modern sequencers have a capacity of more than 15 billion base pairs per run, a maximum read length of more than 600 base pairs, and the ability to analyze up to 96 samples per run [83]. One significant application of NGS technology is whole-genome sequencing (WGS). This technique, which sequences an organism's entire genome, has revolutionized the prediction of antibiotic resistance merely based on point mutations identified on target genes [35]. Furthermore, it enables the detection of novel genetic mutations in clinical isolates, which addresses the limitations of conventional PCR-based assays that can only detect well-known and prevalent mutations. The applicability of WGS extends beyond detecting novel resistance-related mutations in clarithromycin and levofloxacin [36, 84], reaching also to metronidazole [85] and amoxicillin [36, 86]. A study conducted recently in Shenzhen, China, discovered a novel Gln31Arg mutation in the *fliJ* gene in both clarithromycin- and levofloxacin-resistant *H. pylori* strains, and a Ser176Thr/Ala mutation in the *cheA* gene in levofloxacin-resistant strains [84]. Another study in China discovered new mutations in metronidazole-resistant *H. pylori* strains, specifically N118K in *Fur*, Q24K in *Ribf*, and K219Q/N and H705fs in *Omp11* [85]. Two other studies revealed a total of seven novel hypothetical genotypes in *pbp1A*, potentially contributing to amoxicillin resistance [36, 86]. The identification of new candidate genes might offer a better genotypic-phenotypic correlation than currently known genes, enhancing our understanding and management of resistance.

The accuracy of NGS in predicting antibiotic resistance has been found to be satisfactory and largely equivalent to culture-based methodologies, which has been widely accepted as the gold standard for AST. Hulten et al. have illustrated a strong concordance between NGS and agar dilution methods with both clinical isolates and FFPE gastric biopsies, in particular for clarithromycin ($k = 0.900$ and $k = 0.812$ respectively, $p < 0.01$) and levofloxacin ($k = 0.782$ and $k = 0.750$ respectively, $p < 0.01$), albeit less satisfactory for metronidazole and amoxicillin [87]. Building upon these findings, Moss et al. have delved deeper into the accuracy of NGS in predicting antibiotic resistance in stool samples. They found a 91.4% concordance rate between the results from stool samples and those from FFPE gastric biopsies, and a 92.2% concordance rate with fresh gastric specimens [88]. The agreement between stool and fresh gastric samples was substantial for clarithromycin ($k = 0.94$), levofloxacin ($k = 0.88$) and metronidazole ($k = 0.89$). These results highlight the advantage of NGS over conventional PCR assays, which may not be sensitive enough when performed on stool samples, thus positioning NGS as a potentially robust, non-invasive tool for AST.

However, NGS is not without its limitations. Concern about the potential inaccuracy of WGS when applied to gastric biopsies was raised due to the predominance of human DNA and the relatively low content of bacterial DNA [36, 89, 90]. As a result, careful selection and application of appropriate DNA extraction methods are critical. Moreover, the genetic makeup of an organism and the actual observable traits may not always correlate. This discrepancy necessitates further research to validate the predictive accuracy of new genotypes identified by NGS. Such verification can be done using phenotypic outcomes and clinical observations or by retrospectively analyzing the sequencing data [37, 91, 92]. Moreover, current evidence on the accuracy of NGS or WGS in predicting antibiotic resistance mainly lies on clarithromycin, levofloxacin, amoxicillin, and metronidazole. Studies on other antibiotics like tetracycline and rifabutin are limited by small sample sizes due to the low prevalence of antibiotic resistance [35, 87]. Therefore, more comprehensive studies featuring broader gene coverage, larger sample sizes, and multi-center designs spanning different geographical regions are warranted. To facilitate the analysis and application of NGS data in routine clinical practice, there is also a pressing need for the development of standardized, user-friendly computational software and tools [36, 37].

Molecular-based methods provide several advantages over culture-based approaches. They offer a higher degree of standardization and reproducibility, which provides the opportunity for rapid analysis and enables same-day diagnosis. It is more cost-effective as multiple samples can be tested together, and evaluation is simpler without culture. Culture and susceptibility testing require fresh or frozen gastric biopsies. Molecular testing can be performed on the same material and, in addition, can utilize specimens that do not require immediate processing or that are obtained non-invasively [63], including formalin-fixed paraffin-embedded (FFPE) gastric biopsy samples, stool samples, or even gastric juice [37]. Furthermore, molecular test has the advantage over culture-based tests in detecting heteroresistance, which is particularly important in genetic clarithromycin resistance. De Francesco has reported that *H. pylori* infection was cured less frequently in patients with pure resistant strains (46%) than in those infected with hetero-resistant strains (78.5%) or susceptible strains (94.5%) [93].

However, one shoe does not fit all. It must be noted that the majority of molecular tests do not detect resistance based on uncommon genetic mechanisms. Rare mutations within the *rrl* and *gyrA* gene regions, resistances of *H. pylori* strains that lie outside the *rrl* and *gyrA* genes, or other possible mechanisms of clarithromycin and quinolone resistance should also be considered. Also, molecular-based tests cannot distinguish between live and dead cells [94]. Despite the fact that NGS may detect uncommon mutations, the correlation and significance between genotypic resistance and clinical outcomes are yet to be verified. Therefore, results from phenotypic AST approaches are considered more reliable in general, and it was still the gold standard in detecting antibiotic resistance in the current guidelines.

4. Antibiotic stewardship in the treatment of *Helicobacter pylori* infection

The emergence of antibiotic resistance to *H. pylori* is attributed to subtherapeutic levels of an antibiotic, which promotes the survival and natural selection of resistant strains [37]. Antibiotic stewardship is increasingly recognized as a solution to this problem. A series of measures have been advocated to emphasize the judicious use of antibiotics, to encourage the selection of optimal treatment regimens, and to guarantee sustainable access to antibiotics for those who require them [53, 95, 96].

4.1 Issues of the "better-than approach" in *H. pylori* treatment and research

Traditional methods for the treatment of *H. pylori* adopted a trial-and-error approach in which treatment regimens are chosen based on their relative effectiveness compared to conventional empirical regimens, rather than on the absolute cure rate [53, 96]. The conventional "better-than" approach used in clinical trials poses a concern. In cases where none of the treatment arms reach the optimal success rate as defined by antibiotic stewardship, the value of the trial may be compromised [96]. Ethical issues might also arise, as participants may not be informed of potentially suboptimal eradication rates, which have been anticipated based on previous experience [16, 96–98].

Furthermore, overemphasizing relative comparisons in meta-analyses may potentially skew the results, given the inherent heterogeneity among the included clinical trials, such as geographical variations in resistance patterns [96]. Antibiotic stewardship encourages a shift toward therapies with reliably high cure rates [53].

4.2 Susceptibility-guided therapy vs. empirical therapy in achieving antibiotic stewardship

The core principle of antibiotic stewardship is that antibiotics should only be employed to which the bacteria show susceptibility. To achieve an optimal efficacy, treatment regimen should either be guided directly based on AST or indirectly based on test-of-cure results. Yet, the customary empirical therapies employed by physicians in treating *H. pylori* often do not reflect the latest knowledge of local antibiotic resistance patterns, likely due to the unavailability of such data or its delay in dissemination to clinicians. Five meta-analyses have demonstrated that susceptibility-guided therapy (SGT) outperforms empirical regimens in first-line treatment [99–103]. However, it should be noted that these studies exhibited substantial heterogeneity. The differences might not be statistically significant when each empirical regimen is scrutinized independently. The most recent meta-analysis revealed that SGT, by either culture- or PCR-based method, outperformed the empirical clarithromycin-containing triple therapy as a first-line treatment. This was proven in areas with high clarithromycin resistance (>20%) (RR: 1.13, 95% CI: 1.03–1.25), as well as in regions with low clarithromycin resistance (RR: 1.24, 95% CI: 1.15, 1.32) [100]. However, no significant difference was noted in second- or third-line treatments, nor in first-line quadruple therapy [100]. With regard to NGS, recent evidence shows that treatment derived from the routine evaluation of mutations associated with antibiotic resistance using NGS on gastric biopsies offered 4.4 times greater odds of eradication compared to regimens adopted from recommendations provided by NGS-based susceptibility testing reports [104]. However, comparative studies on NGS using other samples, such as stool, are sparse.

The cost-effectiveness of a susceptibility-guided strategy is also an important consideration in *H. pylori* eradication. Much like the cases with efficacy, studies evaluating the cost-effectiveness of susceptibility-guided strategies to empirical treatments have not reached a consensus [64]. Although the continuous refinement of molecular-based methods holds promising results in reducing costs compared to culture-based testing, further studies are necessary to substantiate this claim [7, 105]. Two Korean studies reported that dual priming oligonucleotide (DPO)-PCR-based SGT would only be more cost-effective than empirical triple therapy if the eradication rate of the latter drops below 75–80% [106, 107]. Nonetheless, a study from Korea observed lower total medical costs for SGT as compared to empirical treatments, including triple therapy, sequential therapy, and BQT. The cost of implementing PCR-based SGT in these studies ranges between USD$90.3 [108] and USD$503.5 [109]. The integration of NGS in the design of SGT for routine clinical practice is currently impeded by several factors, including the need for specialized machinery, software, capability in managing extensive genomic data, and personnel trained in the operation of such systems. These collectively contribute to the high cost of NGS, which can reach up to USD$2000–3000 per sample merely for pathogen detection alone [110]. Therefore, routine NGS usage may not be feasible in the short term due to these financial considerations.

It may be conceivable that empirical regimens given according to updated local antibiotic susceptibility patterns are more cost-effective than SGT. Nevertheless, it is essential to continually monitor the performance of these empirical regimens, ensuring the up-to-date adaptation to the ever-changing antibiotic susceptibility patterns.

4.3 Measures to achieve antibiotic stewardship in *H. pylori* treatment

Routine analysis of clinical records comprising diagnosis, treatment, and tests in confirmation of treatment success is an indirect way to evaluate antibiotic susceptibility [53, 96, 111]. Despite the economic advantage and simplicity, such measure is not frequently utilized. The most recent Maastricht VI Florence consensus report has recommended the routine use of susceptibility tests, even before prescribing first-line treatment, with respect to antibiotic stewardship [7]. This recommendation sparks a contrast to earlier guidelines, which suggested that AST was only necessary for patients with failed eradication attempt [112]. Given that molecular methods for AST are increasingly more accessible and affordable, the ultimate goal of shifting toward personalized medicine is one step forward. This individualized strategy aims to maximize eradication rates and minimize the use of inappropriate antibiotics [53, 96, 113].

Implementing antibiotic stewardship in the treatment of *H. pylori* demands a concerted effort from multiple stakeholders. The study showed that compliance was the factor most associated with eradication rates across all evaluated treatment regimens [17]. The importance of drug compliance must be emphasized to patients by their physicians during consultations or by educational campaigns. Physicians should also receive education on the latest trends in antibiotic resistance patterns and relevant guidelines regarding antibiotic use. Local healthcare authorities should take the initiative to establish antibiotic stewardship programs that incorporate routine AST in clinical settings, monitor antibiotic prescriptions and resistance patterns, and provide treatment guidelines tailored to their local resistance pattern. At the international level, consensus reports and guidelines play a vital role in promoting antibiotic stewardship measures and providing evidence-based treatment recommendations. Existing antibiotic surveillance programs, both locally and internationally, should include *H. pylori* if it is not already incorporated. The collective contributions from all stakeholders are essential to ensure the successful application of antibiotic stewardship in the treatment of *H. pylori* infection.

5. Adjuncts and new agents in *H. pylori* eradication

The changing profile of *H. pylori* antibiotic resistance greatly affects the efficacy of empirical therapies. Despite the appropriate eradication regimens, persistent infection was found in around 10% of patients. Continuous development of better treatment regimens and discovery of novel agents against *H. pylori* infection are required [114].

Recently, vonoprazan, a potassium-competitive acid blocker (P-CAB), which demonstrates greater gastric acid-suppressive potency than PPIs, has been incorporated into eradication treatments. Stronger acid suppression by keeping the gastric acidity at a pH greater than 6 is the key in *H. pylori* eradication. Such a microenvironment promotes bacterial growth and renders antibiotics to be more efficient. Several clinical trials conducted in Asia have highlighted the potential of vonoprazan in achieving eradication rates of over 90% [115–122]. As such, Maastricht VI consensus has recommended using P-CAB–antimicrobial combination treatments in patients with evidence of antimicrobial-resistant infections.

Probiotics also play a role as an add-on to eradication. It can enhance antibiotic activity and inhibit resistance by altering gastric microenvironment pH, modulating immunity, producing antioxidants, and affecting *H. pylori* colonization [123]. Probiotics, mainly *Lactobacillus*, *Saccharomyces boulardii*, or *Bacillus clausii*, were studied. A meta-analysis found that patients treated with probiotics had a higher eradication rate than those not treated with probiotics (80.3% vs. 72.2%). A growing number of systematic reviews and meta-analyses have also observed decreased side effects, such as diarrhea caused by *H. pylori* eradication therapies [123].

Few novel drugs have been proposed to treat *H.* pylori infection. Finafloxacin, a novel fluoroquinolone, was shown to have high antimicrobial efficacy against *H. pylori* in an acidic environment at pH = 5 [124]. Flavodoxin inhibitor, an agent that targets the unique flavodoxin component of an essential metabolic pathway of *H. pylori*, was shown to have bactericidal activity against *H. pylori* cells [125]. Further evaluation is needed to ensure the safety and adequate effectiveness of these agents.

Anti-*H. pylori* vaccine development may be a new strategy to reduce the prevalence of *H. pylori* infection. A phase III randomized controlled trial reported a satisfying result of vaccination success in 71.8% of Chinese children within the first year [126]. However, more data is needed to support its use where epitope mapping, determination of antigen choice, genomic approach, and safety assessment have to be evaluated.

6. Conclusion

To combat the growing threat of *H. pylori* resistance, there is an imperative need for a multifaceted approach, including the development of new antibiotics, the implementation of stewardship programs to prevent overuse, the improvement of

	Prevalence	**Resistance mechanisms**
Clarithromycin	Europe: 18% America: 10% [28] Southeast Asia: 10% [28] African: 29.2% [31]	Point mutations in 23S rRNA gene Increased antibiotic efflux Alteration of outer membrane proteins
Metronidazole	Europe: 32%. America: 23% China: 87.8% Oceania: 50% [127]	Mutations in metronidazole-reducing enzymes coding genes, mainly RdxA coding gene, *frxA* or *fdxB* gene Increased antibiotic efflux
Levofloxacin	Europe: 20% [33] America: 14% [28] Asia: 18% [128] Africa: 17.4% [31]	Point mutations in quinolones resistance-determining region (QRDR)
Amoxicillin	Europe: 0.4% [33] Asia: 3% [128] Africa: 72.6% [31]	Mutations in the penicillin-binding proteins Increased antibiotic efflux Production of β-lactamase
Tetracycline	Europe: <1% [33] America: 0.87% [30] China: 1.18% [129]	Point mutations in 16S ribosomal primary binding site Increased antibiotic efflux

Table 1.
Resistance rate and resistance mechanism of antibiotics commonly used in Helicobacter pylori *eradication therapies.*

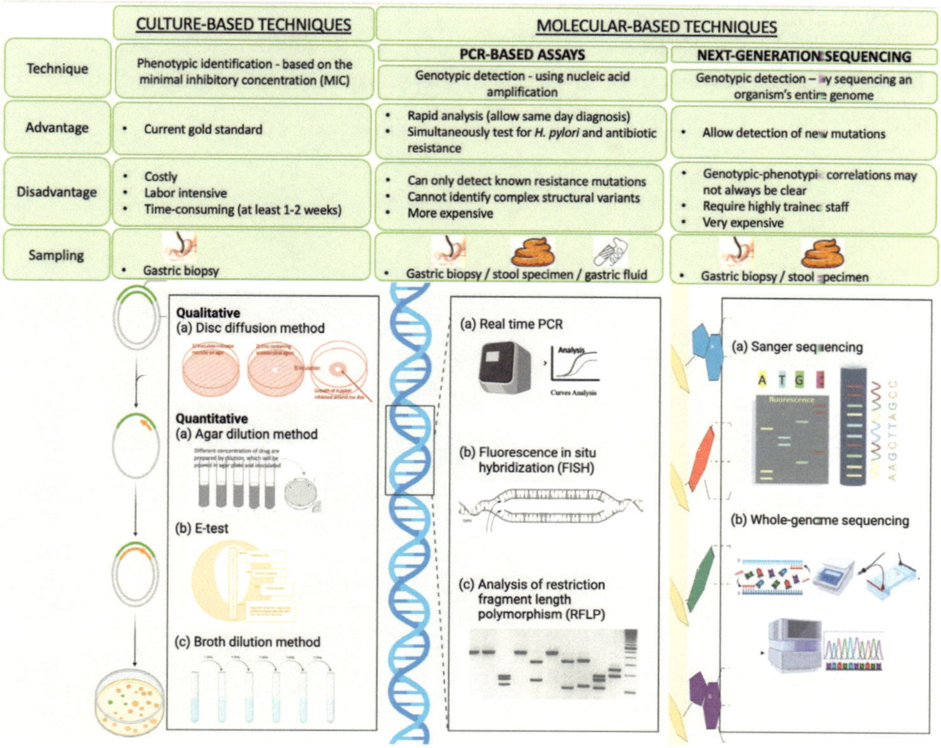

Figure 1.
Comparison of culture-based and molecular-based antibiotic susceptibility testing (AST) methods.

diagnostic methods to tailor therapy to individual resistance profiles, and increased funding for research in alternative therapies and the development of standardized, user-friendly computational software and tools. The implementation of antibiotic stewardship is crucial to maintaining the efficacy of current treatment protocols. A key aspect of antibiotic stewardship involves carrying out antibiotic susceptibility testing prior to the initiation of empirical treatment. The major technological strides have paved the way for molecular-based sequencing techniques, enabling swift and convenient detection of antibiotic resistance. In particular, stool-based molecular tests may prove to be an integral part of routine clinical practice going forward due to their ease of use and prompt results. Additionally, WGS holds the potential to uncover novel genetic mutations related to antibiotic resistance. However, these findings must be substantiated through rigorous validation studies to ensure their clinical relevance and accuracy (**Table 1** and **Figure 1**).

Funding

This research received no external funding.

Conflicts of interest

The authors declare no conflict of interest.

Data availability statement

No new data were created or analyzed in this study.

Author details

Lok Ka Lam[1] and Ka Shing Cheung[1,2]*

1 Department of Medicine, School of Clinical Medicine, The University of Hong Kong, Queen Mary Hospital, Hong Kong, China

2 Department of Medicine, The University of Hong Kong-Shenzhen Hospital, Shenzhen, China

*Address all correspondence to: cks634@hku.hk

References

[1] Graham DY. Can therapy even be denied for Helicobacter pylori infection? Gastroenterology. 1997;**113**:S113-S117

[2] Gloeckler Ries LA, Reichman ME, Lewis DR, et al. Cancer survival and incidence from the Surveillance, Epidemiology, and End Results (SEER) program. The Oncologist. 2003;**8**:541-552

[3] Graham DY. The only good Helicobacter pylori is a dead *Helicobacter pylori*. Lancet. 1997;**350**:70-71; author reply 72

[4] Correa P. Human gastric carcinogenesis: A multistep and multifactorial process—first American Cancer Society award lecture on cancer epidemiology and prevention. Cancer Research. 1992;**52**:6735-6740

[5] Sung H, Ferlay J, Siegel RL, et al. Global cancer statistics 2020: GLOBOCAN estimates of incidence and mortality worldwide for 36 cancers in 185 countries. CA: A Cancer Journal for Clinicians. 2021;**71**:209-249

[6] Sugano K, Tack J, Kuipers EJ, et al. Kyoto global consensus report on *Helicobacter pylori* gastritis. Gut. 2015;**64**:1353-1367

[7] Malfertheiner P, Megraud F, Rokkas T, et al. Management of *Helicobacter pylori* infection: The Maastricht VI/Florence consensus report. Gut. 2022;**71**:1724-1762

[8] Boltin D, Niv Y, Schutte K, et al. Review: Helicobacter pylori and non-malignant upper gastrointestinal diseases. Helicobacter. 2019;**24** (Suppl. 1):e12637

[9] Hentschel E, Brandstatter G, Dragosics B, et al. Effect of ranitidine and amoxicillin plus metronidazole on the eradication of *Helicobacter pylori* and the recurrence of duodenal ulcer. The New England Journal of Medicine. 1993;**328**:308-312

[10] Lee YC, Liou JM, Wu MS, et al. Eradication of *Helicobacter pylori* to prevent gastroduodenal diseases: Hitting more than one bird with the same stone. Therapeutic Advances in Gastroenterology. 2008;**1**:111-120

[11] Lee YC, Chiang TH, Chou CK, et al. Association between *Helicobacter pylori* eradication and gastric cancer incidence: A systematic review and meta-analysis. Gastroenterology. 2016;**150**(1113-1124):e5

[12] Chiang TH, Chang WJ, Chen SL, et al. Mass eradication of Helicobacter pylori to reduce gastric cancer incidence and mortality: A long-term cohort study on Matsu Islands. Gut. 2021;**70**:243-250

[13] Leung WK, Wong IOL, Cheung KS, et al. Effects of *Helicobacter pylori* treatment on incidence of gastric cancer in older individuals. Gastroenterology. 2018;**155**:67-75

[14] Chey WD, Wong BC. Practice parameters committee of the American College of G. American College of Gastroenterology guideline on the management of *Helicobacter pylori* infection. The American Journal of Gastroenterology. 2007;**102**:1808-1825

[15] Howden CW, Hunt RH. Guidelines for the management of *Helicobacter pylori* infection. Ad Hoc Committee on Practice Parameters of the American College of Gastroenterology. The American Journal of Gastroenterology. 1998;**93**:2330-2338

[16] Graham DY, Fischbach L. *Helicobacter pylori* treatment in the era of increasing antibiotic resistance. Gut. 2010;**59**:1143-1153

[17] Nyssen OP, Bordin D, Tepes B, et al. European registry on *Helicobacter pylori* management (Hp-EuReg): Patterns and trends in first-line empirical eradication prescription and outcomes of 5 years and 21 533 patients. Gut. 2021;**70**:40-54

[18] Sun Q, Liang X, Zheng Q, et al. High efficacy of 14-day triple therapy-based, bismuth-containing quadruple therapy for initial *Helicobacter pylori* eradication. Helicobacter. 2010;**15**:233-238

[19] Hsu PI, Chen KY, Tai WC, et al. Hybrid, high-dose dual and bismuth quadruple therapies for first-line treatment of *Helicobacter pylori* infection in Taiwan: A multicenter, open-label, randomized trial. The American Journal of Gastroenterology. 2023;**118**:1184-1195

[20] Chey WD, Leontiadis GI, Howden CW, et al. ACG clinical guideline: Treatment of *Helicobacter pylori* Infection. The American Journal of Gastroenterology. 2017;**112**:212-239

[21] Fallone CA, Chiba N, van Zanten SV, et al. The Toronto consensus for the treatment of *Helicobacter pylori* infection in adults. Gastroenterology. 2016;**151**: 51-69 e14

[22] Hulten KG, Lamberth LB, Kalfus IN, et al. National and regional US antibiotic resistance to *Helicobacter pylori*: Lessons from a clinical trial. Gastroenterology. 2021;**161**:342-344 e1

[23] Chen J, Li P, Huang Y, et al. Primary antibiotic resistance of *Helicobacter pylori* in Different regions of China: A systematic review and meta-analysis. Pathogens. 2022;7:11

[24] Ji Y, Lu H. Meta-analysis: High-dose vs. low-dose metronidazole-containing therapies for *Helicobacter pylori* eradication treatment. PLoS One. 2018;**13**:e0189888

[25] Losurdo G, Leandro G, Principi M, et al. Sequential vs. prolonged 14-day triple therapy for *Helicobacter pylori* eradication: The meta-analysis may be influenced by 'geographical weighting'. International Journal of Clinical Practice. 2015;**69**:1112-1120

[26] Losurdo G, Pricci M, De Bellis M, et al. Effect of metronidazole resistance on *Helicobacter pylori* eradication regimens. Journal of Digestive Diseases. 2022;**23**:561-567

[27] Gerding DN. The search for good antimicrobial stewardship. Joint Commission Journal on Quality Improvement. 2001;**27**:403-404

[28] Savoldi A, Carrara E, Graham DY, et al. Prevalence of antibiotic resistance in *Helicobacter pylori*: A systematic review and meta-analysis in World Health Organization Regions. Gastroenterology. 2018;**155**:1372-1382 e17

[29] Hong TC, El-Omar EM, Kuo YT, et al. Primary antibiotic resistance of *Helicobacter pylori* in the Asia-Pacific region between 1990 and 2022: An updated systematic review and meta-analysis. The Lancet Gastroenterology & Hepatology. 2024;**9**:56-67

[30] Ho JJC, Navarro M, Sawyer K, et al. *Helicobacter pylori* antibiotic resistance in the United States between 2011 and 2021: A systematic review and meta-analysis. The American Journal of Gastroenterology. 2022;**117**:1221-1230

[31] Jaka H, Rhee JA, Ostlundh L, et al. The magnitude of antibiotic resistance to Helicobacter pylori in Africa and

identified mutations which confer resistance to antibiotics: Systematic review and meta-analysis. BMC Infectious Diseases. 2018;**18**:193

[32] Camargo CM, García A, Riquelme A, et al. The problem of *Helicobacter pylori* resistance to antibiotics: A systematic review in Latin America. Official Journal of the American College of Gastroenterology| ACG. 2014;**109**:485-495

[33] Bujanda L, Nyssen OP, Vaira D, et al. Antibiotic resistance prevalence and trends in patients infected with *Helicobacter pylori* in the period 2013-2020: Results of the European Registry on H. pylori Management (Hp-EuReg). Antibiotics (Basel). 2021;**20**:10

[34] Tuan VP, Narith D, Tshibangu-Kabamba E, et al. A next-generation sequencing-based approach to identify genetic determinants of antibiotic resistance in Cambodian *Helicobacter pylori* clinical isolates. Journal of Clinical Medicine. 2019;**8**:8

[35] Lauener FN, Imkamp F, Lehours P, et al. Genetic determinants and prediction of antibiotic resistance phenotypes in *Helicobacter pylori*. Journal of Clinical Medicine. 2019;**8**:8

[36] Tshibangu-Kabamba E, Ngoma-Kisoko PJ, Tuan VP, et al. Next-generation sequencing of the whole bacterial genome for tracking molecular insight into the broad-spectrum antimicrobial resistance of *Helicobacter pylori* clinical isolates from the Democratic Republic of Congo. Microorganisms. 2020;**8**:8

[37] Tshibangu-Kabamba E, Yamaoka Y. *Helicobacter pylori* infection and antibiotic resistance - From biology to clinical implications. Nature Reviews. Gastroenterology & Hepatology. 2021;**18**:613-629

[38] Hu Y, Zhang M, Lu B, et al. *Helicobacter pylori* and antibiotic resistance, a continuing and intractable problem. Helicobacter. 2016;**21**:349-363

[39] Gong Y, Yuan Y. Resistance mechanisms of *Helicobacter pylori* and its dual target precise therapy. Critical Reviews in Microbiology. 2018;**44**:371-392

[40] Versalovic J, Shortridge D, Kibler K, et al. Mutations in 23S rRNA are associated with clarithromycin resistance in *Helicobacter pylori*. Antimicrobial Agents and Chemotherapy. 1996;**40**:477-480

[41] Puah SM, Goh KL, Ng HK, et al. Current status of *Helicobacter pylori* resistance to Clarithromycin and Levofloxacin in Malaysia-findings from a molecular based study. PeerJ. 2021;**9**:e11518

[42] Jeong JY, Mukhopadhyay AK, Akada JK, et al. Roles of FrxA and RdxA nitroreductases of *Helicobacter pylori* in susceptibility and resistance to metronidazole. Journal of Bacteriology. 2001;**183**:5155-5162

[43] Rimbara E, Noguchi N, Kawai T, et al. Fluoroquinolone resistance in *Helicobacter pylori*: Role of mutations at position 87 and 91 of GyrA on the level of resistance and identification of a resistance conferring mutation in GyrB. Helicobacter. 2012;**17**:36-42

[44] Rimbara E, Noguchi N, Kawai T, et al. Mutations in penicillin-binding proteins 1, 2 and 3 are responsible for amoxicillin resistance in *Helicobacter pylori*. The Journal of Antimicrobial Chemotherapy. 2008;**61**:995-998

[45] Lin Y, Shao Y, Yan J, et al. Antibiotic resistance in *Helicobacter pylori*: From potential biomolecular mechanisms

to clinical practice. Journal of Clinical Laboratory Analysis. 2023;**37**:e24885

[46] Megraud F, Bruyndonckx R, Coenen S, et al. *Helicobacter pylori* resistance to antibiotics in Europe in 2018 and its relationship to antibiotic consumption in the community. Gut. 2021;**70**:1815-1822

[47] Wang D, Guo Q, Yuan Y, et al. The antibiotic resistance of *Helicobacter pylori* to five antibiotics and influencing factors in an area of China with a high risk of gastric cancer. BMC Microbiology. 2019;**19**:152

[48] Tang X, Wang Z, Shen Y, et al. Antibiotic resistance patterns of *Helicobacter pylori* strains isolated from the Tibet Autonomous Region, China. BMC Microbiology. 2022;**22**:196

[49] Cosme A, Lizasoan J, Montes M, et al. Antimicrobial susceptibility-guided therapy versus empirical concomitant therapy for eradication of *Helicobacter pylori* in a region with high rate of clarithromycin resistance. Helicobacter. 2016;**21**:29-34

[50] Sarem M, Corti R. Role of *Helicobacter pylori* coccoid forms in infection and recrudescence. Gastroenterología y Hepatología. 2016;**39**:28-35

[51] Kadkhodaei S, Siavoshi F, Akbari NK. Mucoid and coccoid *Helicobacter pylori* with fast growth and antibiotic resistance. Helicobacter. 2020;**25**:e12678

[52] Andersson DI, Nicoloff H, Hjort K. Mechanisms and clinical relevance of bacterial heteroresistance. Nature Reviews. Microbiology. 2019;**17**:479-496

[53] Graham DY, Liou JM. Primer for development of guidelines for *Helicobacter pylori* therapy using antimicrobial stewardship. Clinical Gastroenterology and Hepatology. 2022;**20**:973-983 e1

[54] Gerrits MM, van Vliet AH, Kuipers EJ, et al. *Helicobacter pylori* and antimicrobial resistance: Molecular mechanisms and clinical implications. The Lancet Infectious Diseases. 2006;**6**:699-709

[55] Arslan N, Yilmaz O, Demiray-Gurbuz E. Importance of antimicrobial susceptibility testing for the management of eradication in *Helicobacter pylori* infection. World Journal of Gastroenterology. 2017;**23**:2854-2869

[56] Grignon B, Tankovic J, Megraud F, et al. Validation of diffusion methods for macrolide susceptibility testing of *Helicobacter pylori*. Microbial Drug Resistance. 2002;**8**:61-66

[57] Best LM, Haldane DJ, Keelan M, et al. Multilaboratory comparison of proficiencies in susceptibility testing of *Helicobacter pylori* and correlation between agar dilution and E test methods. Antimicrobial Agents and Chemotherapy. 2003;**47**:3138-3144

[58] Megraud F, Hazell S, Glupczynski Y. Antibiotic susceptibility and resistance. In: HLT M, Mendz GL, Hazell SL, editors. *Helicobacter pylori*: Physiology and Genetics. Washington (DC); 2001

[59] Phan TN, Tran VH, Tran TN, et al. Antimicrobial resistance in *Helicobacter pylori*: Current situation and management strategy in Vietnam. Journal of Infection in Developing Countries. 2015;**9**:609-613

[60] Thung I, Aramin H, Vavinskaya V, et al. Review article: The global emergence of *Helicobacter pylori* antibiotic resistance. Alimentary Pharmacology & Therapeutics. 2016;**43**:514-533

[61] Boyanova L. Comparative evaluation of two methods for testing metronidazole susceptibility of *Helicobacter pylori* in routine practice. Diagnostic Microbiology and Infectious Disease. 1999;**35**:33-36

[62] Graham DY, Moss SF. Antimicrobial susceptibility testing for *Helicobacter pylori* is now widely available: When, how, why. American Journal of Gastroenterology. 2022;**117**:524-528

[63] Pohl D, Keller PM, Bordier V, et al. Review of current diagnostic methods and advances in *Helicobacter pylori* diagnostics in the era of next generation sequencing. World Journal of Gastroenterology. 2019;**25**:4629-4660

[64] Gisbert JP. Empirical or susceptibility-guided treatment for *Helicobacter pylori* infection? A comprehensive review. Therapeutic Advances in Gastroenterology. 2020;**13**:1756284820968736

[65] Megraud F. Resistance of *Helicobacter pylori* to antibiotics. Alimentary Pharmacology & Therapeutics. 1997;**11**(Suppl. 1):43-53

[66] Francesco V, Zullo A, Manta R, et al. Culture-based antibiotic susceptibility testing for *Helicobacter pylori* infection: A systematic review. Annals of Gastroenterology. 2022;**35**:127-134

[67] Fernandez-Caso B, Miqueleiz A, Valdez VB, et al. Are molecular methods helpful for the diagnosis of *Helicobacter pylori* infection and for the prediction of its antimicrobial resistance? Frontiers in Microbiology. 2022;**13**:962063

[68] Ierardi E, Giorgio F, Losurdo G, et al. How antibiotic resistances could change *Helicobacter pylori* treatment: A matter of geography? World Journal of Gastroenterology. 2013;**19**:8168-8180

[69] Redondo JJ, Keller PM, Zbinden R, et al. A novel RT-PCR for the detection of Helicobacter pylori and identification of clarithromycin resistance mediated by mutations in the 23S rRNA gene. Diagnostic Microbiology and Infectious Disease. 2018;**90**:1-6

[70] Schabereiter-Gurtner C, Hirschl AM, Dragosics B, et al. Novel real-time PCR assay for detection of Helicobacter pylori infection and simultaneous clarithromycin susceptibility testing of stool and biopsy specimens. Journal of Clinical Microbiology. 2004;**42**:4512-4518

[71] Beckman E, Saracino I, Fiorini G, et al. A novel stool PCR test for *Helicobacter pylori* may predict clarithromycin resistance and eradication of infection at a high rate. Journal of Clinical Microbiology. 2017;**55**:2400-2405

[72] Lottspeich C, Schwarzer A, Panthel K, et al. Evaluation of the novel *Helicobacter pylori* ClariRes real-time PCR assay for detection and clarithromycin susceptibility testing of *H. pylori* in stool specimens from symptomatic children. Journal of Clinical Microbiology. 2007;**45**:1718-1722

[73] Vecsei A, Innerhofer A, Binder C, et al. Stool polymerase chain reaction for *Helicobacter pylori* detection and clarithromycin susceptibility testing in children. Clinical Gastroenterology and Hepatology. 2010;**8**:309-312

[74] Scaletsky IC, Aranda KR, Garcia GT, et al. Application of real-time PCR stool assay for *Helicobacter pylori* detection and clarithromycin susceptibility testing in Brazilian children. Helicobacter. 2011;**16**:311-315

[75] Megraud F, Lehours P. *Helicobacter pylori* detection and antimicrobial

susceptibility testing. Clinical Microbiology Reviews. 2007;**20**:280-322

[76] Patel SK, Pratap CB, Jain AK, et al. Diagnosis of *Helicobacter pylori*: What should be the gold standard? World Journal of Gastroenterology. 2014;**20**:12847-12859

[77] Ciesielska U, Jagoda E, Marciniak Z. Value of PCR technique in detection of *Helicobacter pylori* in paraffin-embedded material. Folia Histochemica et Cytobiologica. 2002;**40**:129-130

[78] Wang L, Lai JX, Si YT, et al. Quantitative polymerase chain reaction (qPCR)-based rapid diagnosis of *Helicobacter pylori* infection and antibiotic resistance. Journal of Visualized Experiments. 2023

[79] Jia-Wei Tang FL, Liu X, et al. Detection of *Helicobacter pylori* infection in human gastric fluid through surface-enhanced raman spectroscopy coupled with machine learning algorithms. Laboratory Investigation. 2023;**104**:104

[80] Han X, Yu X, Gao X, et al. Quantitative PCR of string-test collected gastric material: A feasible approach to detect *Helicobacter pylori* and its resistance against clarithromycin and levofloxacin for susceptibility-guided therapy. Helicobacter. 2023;**28**:e12985

[81] Al-Shuhaib MBS, Hashim HO. Mastering DNA chromatogram analysis in Sanger sequencing for reliable clinical analysis. Journal, Genetic Engineering & Biotechnology. 2023;**21**:115

[82] Slatko BE, Gardner AF, Ausubel FM. Overview of next-generation sequencing technologies. Current Protocols in Molecular Biology. 2018;**122**:e59

[83] Barba M, Czosnek H, Hadidi A. Historical perspective, development and applications of next-generation sequencing in plant virology. Viruses. 2014;**6**:106-136

[84] Lyu T, Cheung KS, Deng Z, et al. Whole genome sequencing reveals novel genetic mutations of *Helicobacter pylori* associating with resistance to clarithromycin and levofloxacin. Helicobacter. 2023;**28**:e12972

[85] Zhou Y, Zhong Z, Hu S, et al. A survey of *Helicobacter pylori* antibiotic-resistant genotypes and strain lineages by whole-genome sequencing in China. Antimicrobial Agents and Chemotherapy. 2022;**66**:e0218821

[86] Fauzia KA, Aftab H, Tshibangu-Kabamba E, et al. Mutations related to antibiotics resistance in *Helicobacter pylori* clinical isolates from Bangladesh. Antibiotics (Basel). 2023;**12**:12

[87] Hulten KG, Genta RM, Kalfus IN, et al. Comparison of culture with antibiogram to next-generation sequencing using bacterial isolates and formalin-fixed, paraffin-embedded gastric biopsies. Gastroenterology. 2021;**161**:1433-1442 e2

[88] Moss SF, Dang LP, Chua D, et al. Comparable results of *Helicobacter pylori* antibiotic resistance testing of stools vs gastric biopsies using next-generation sequencing. Gastroenterology. 2022;**162**:2095-2097 e2

[89] Egli K, Wagner K, Keller PM, et al. Comparison of the diagnostic performance of qPCR, sanger sequencing, and whole-genome sequencing in determining clarithromycin and levofloxacin resistance in *Helicobacter pylori*. Frontiers in Cellular and Infection Microbiology. 2020;**10**:596371

[90] Hendriksen RS, Bortolaia V, Tate H, et al. Using genomics to track global

antimicrobial resistance. Frontiers in Public Health. 2019;**7**:242

[91] Yusibova M, Hasman H, Clausen P, et al. CRHP Finder, a webtool for the detection of clarithromycin resistance in *Helicobacter pylori* from whole-genome sequencing data. Helicobacter. 2020;**25**:e12752

[92] Saracino IM, Pavoni M, Zullo A, et al. Next generation sequencing for the prediction of the antibiotic resistance in *Helicobacter pylori*: A literature review. Antibiotics (Basel). 2021;**10**:10

[93] De Francesco V, Zullo A, Ierardi E, et al. Phenotypic and genotypic *Helicobacter pylori* clarithromycin resistance and therapeutic outcome: Benefits and limits. The Journal of Antimicrobial Chemotherapy. 2010;**65**:327-332

[94] Cangelosi GA, Meschke JS. Dead or alive: Molecular assessment of microbial viability. Applied and Environmental Microbiology. 2014;**80**:5884-5891

[95] Infectious Diseases Society of A. White paper: Recommendations on the conduct of superiority and organism-specific clinical trials of antibacterial agents for the treatment of infections caused by drug-resistant bacterial pathogens. Clinical Infectious Diseases. 2012;**55**:1031-1046

[96] Graham DY. Transitioning of *Helicobacter pylori* therapy from trial and error to antimicrobial stewardship. Antibiotics (Basel). 2020;**9**:9

[97] Graham DY. Efficient identification and evaluation of effective *Helicobacter pylori* therapies. Clinical Gastroenterology and Hepatology. 2009;**7**:145-148

[98] Graham DY. *Helicobacter pylori* eradication therapy research: Ethical issues and description of results. Clinical Gastroenterology and Hepatology. 2010;**8**:1032-1036

[99] Wenzhen Y, Yumin L, Quanlin G, et al. Is antimicrobial susceptibility testing necessary before first-line treatment for *Helicobacter pylori* infection? Meta-analysis of randomized controlled trials. Internal Medicine. 2010;**49**:1103-1109

[100] Nyssen OP, Espada M, Gisbert JP. Empirical vs. susceptibility-guided treatment of *Helicobacter pylori* infection: A systematic review and meta-analysis. Frontiers in Microbiology. 2022;**13**:913436

[101] Gingold-Belfer R, Niv Y, Schmilovitz-Weiss H, et al. Susceptibility-guided versus empirical treatment for *Helicobacter pylori* infection: A systematic review and meta-analysis. Journal of Gastroenterology and Hepatology. 2021;**36**:2649-2658

[102] Lopez-Gongora S, Puig I, Calvet X, et al. Systematic review and meta-analysis: Susceptibility-guided versus empirical antibiotic treatment for *Helicobacter pylori* infection. The Journal of Antimicrobial Chemotherapy. 2015;**70**:2447-2455

[103] Chen H, Dang Y, Zhou X, et al. Tailored therapy versus empiric chosen treatment for *Helicobacter pylori* eradication: A meta-analysis. Medicine (Baltimore). 2016;**95**:e2750

[104] Cummings LC, Hojat LS, Nguyen DC, et al. Tailored treatment based on *Helicobacter pylori* genetic markers of resistance is associated with higher eradication success. The American Journal of Gastroenterology. 2023;**118**:360-363

[105] El-Serag HB, Kao JY, Kanwal F, et al. Houston consensus conference on testing

for *Helicobacter pylori* infection in the United States. Clinical Gastroenterology and Hepatology. 2018;**16**:992-1002 e6

[106] Cho JH, Jeon SR, Kim HG, et al. Cost-effectiveness of a tailored *Helicobacter pylori* eradication strategy based on the presence of a 23S ribosomal RNA point mutation that causes clarithromycin resistance in Korean patients. Journal of Gastroenterology and Hepatology. 2019;**34**:700-706

[107] Gweon TG, Kim JS, Kim BW. An economic modeling study of *Helicobacter pylori* eradication: Comparison of dual priming oligonucleotide-based multiplex polymerase chain reaction and empirical treatment. Gut Liver. 2018;**12**:648-654

[108] Cha B, Bang BW, Shin JB, et al. Bismuth containing quadruple therapy versus tailored therapy as first-line treatments for *Helicobacter pylori* infection in a high clarithromycin resistance area. Scandinavian Journal of Gastroenterology. 2021;**56**:1017-1022

[109] Chang YW, Shin GY, Kim JW, et al. Cost-effectiveness of empirical bismuth-based quadruple therapy and tailored therapy after clarithromycin resistance tests for *Helicobacter pylori* eradication. Digestive Diseases and Sciences. 2022;**67**:1222-1230

[110] Waskito LA, Rezkitha YAA, Vilaichone RK, et al. Antimicrobial resistance profile by metagenomic and metatranscriptomic approach in clinical practice: Opportunity and challenge. Antibiotics (Basel). 2022;**11**:11

[111] Ginnebaugh BD, Baker J, Watts L, et al. S1348 triple therapy for primary treatment of *Helicobacter pylori*: A 19-year U.S. single center experience. Official Journal of the American College of Gastroenterology | ACG. 2020;**115**:115

[112] Malfertheiner P, Megraud F, O'Morain CA, et al. Management of *Helicobacter pylori* infection-the Maastricht V/Florence Consensus Report. Gut. 2017;**66**:6-30

[113] Shiotani A, Roy P, Lu H, et al. Helicobacter pylori diagnosis and therapy in the era of antimicrobial stewardship. Therapeutic Advances in Gastroenterology. 2021;**14**:17562848211064080

[114] Siddique O, Ovalle A, Siddique AS, et al. *Helicobacter pylori* infection: An update for the internist in the age of increasing global antibiotic resistance. The American Journal of Medicine. 2018;**131**:473-479

[115] Bunchorntavakul C, Buranathawornsom A. Randomized clinical trial: 7-day vonoprazan-based versus 14-day omeprazole-based triple therapy for *Helicobacter pylori*. Journal of Gastroenterology and Hepatology. 2021;**36**:3308-3313

[116] Lu L, Wang Y, Ye J, et al. Quadruple therapy with vonoprazan 20 mg daily as a first-line treatment for *Helicobacter pylori* infection: A single-center, open-label, noninferiority, randomized controlled trial. Helicobacter. 2023;**28**:e12940

[117] Maruyama M, Tanaka N, Kubota D, et al. Vonoprazan-based regimen is more useful than PPI-based one as a first-line *Helicobacter pylori* eradication: A randomized controlled trial. Canadian Journal of Gastroenterology & Hepatology. 2017;**2017**:4385161

[118] Murakami K, Sakurai Y, Shiino M, et al. Vonoprazan, a novel potassium-competitive acid blocker, as a component of first-line and second-line triple therapy for Helicobacter pylori eradication: A phase III,

randomised, double-blind study. Gut. 2016;**65**:1439-1446

[119] Hou X, Meng F, Wang J, et al. Vonoprazan non-inferior to lansoprazole in treating duodenal ulcer and eradicating Helicobacter pylori in Asian patients. Journal of Gastroenterology and Hepatology. 2022;**37**:1275-1283

[120] Qian HS, Li WJ, Dang YN, et al. Ten-day vonoprazan-amoxicillin dual therapy as a first-line treatment of *Helicobacter pylori* infection compared with bismuth-containing quadruple therapy. The American Journal of Gastroenterology. 2023;**118**:627-634

[121] Zuberi BF, Ali FS, Rasheed T, et al. Comparison of vonoprazan and amoxicillin dual therapy with standard triple therapy with proton pump inhibitor for *Helicobacter Pylori* eradication: A randomized control trial. Pakistan Journal of Medical Sciences. 2022;**38**:965-969

[122] Huh KY, Chung H, Kim YK, et al. Evaluation of safety and pharmacokinetics of bismuth-containing quadruple therapy with either vonoprazan or lansoprazole for *Helicobacter pylori* eradication. British Journal of Clinical Pharmacology. 2022;**88**:138-144

[123] Gonzalez-Bello C. Antibiotic adjuvants - A strategy to unlock bacterial resistance to antibiotics. Bioorganic & Medicinal Chemistry Letters. 2017;**27**:4221-4228

[124] Lee JW, Kim N, Nam RH, et al. High efficacy of finafloxacin on *Helicobacter pylori* isolates at pH 5.0 compared with that of other fluoroquinolones. Antimicrobial Agents and Chemotherapy. 2015;**59**:7629-7636

[125] Salillas S, Sancho J. Flavodoxins as novel therapeutic targets against *Helicobacter pylori* and other gastric pathogens. International Journal of Molecular Sciences. 2020;**21**:1881

[126] Zeng M, Mao XH, Li JX, et al. Efficacy, safety, and immunogenicity of an oral recombinant *Helicobacter pylori* vaccine in children in China: A randomised, double-blind, placebo-controlled, phase 3 trial. Lancet. 2015;**386**:1457-1464

[127] Schubert JP, Gehlert J, Rayner CK, et al. Antibiotic resistance of *Helicobacter pylori* in Australia and New Zealand: A systematic review and meta-analysis. Journal of Gastroenterology and Hepatology. 2021;**36**:1450-1456

[128] Kuo YT, Liou JM, El-Omar EM, et al. Primary antibiotic resistance in *Helicobacter pylori* in the Asia-Pacific region: A systematic review and meta-analysis. The Lancet Gastroenterology & Hepatology. 2017;**2**:707-715

[129] Zhong Z, Zhang Z, Wang J, et al. A retrospective study of the antibiotic-resistant phenotypes and genotypes of *Helicobacter pylori* strains in China. American Journal of Cancer Research. 2021;**11**:5027-5037

Chapter 6

Helicobacter pylori and Oral Pathology

Isabel Adler, Andrea Muiño, Pablo Rodríguez and Valeria Denninghoff

Abstract

Helicobacter pylori (Hp) is one of the most common infections worldwide, with important implications in gastric pathology. Early diagnosis and treatment are essential for the control and prevention of gastric diseases. The role of Hp in the oral cavity has been investigated and studied for the past 30 years, with a growing interest because oral-oral transmission is one of the main routes. In patients with burning, halitosis, and lingual papillary hypertrophy (BHH) in the oral cavity, the dental plaque and lingual dorsum have been identified as Hp reservoirs for colonization. BHH is suggested as an effective marker for early diagnosis of Hp infection, which should be confirmed by molecular techniques and correlated with gastric involvement.

Keywords: *Helicobacter pylori*, oral pathology, oral-oral transmission, dental plaque, lingual dorsum, burning, halitosis, and lingual papillary hypertrophy (BHH)

1. Introduction

Helicobacter pylori (Hp) is a highly mobile gram-negative, distinctively twisted helix bacterium responsible for the most common chronic bacterial infection in humans, present in all populations and individuals of all ages. This bacterium was discovered by Dr. Barry Marshall and Dr. Robin Warren in 1982, who demonstrated that Hp can cause gastritis, receiving the Nobel Prize in 2005 due to the broad implications of their findings [1].

However, it was observed that the annual reoccurrence rate of Hp after eradication of successful gastric infection was 13% due to oral Hp infection, even in patients with negative urea breath test results, which indicates that the stomach Hp infection was cured in these patients. Reinfection in these patients suggested that the oral cavity is a secondary site for Hp colonization [2]. So, from these findings, three transmission routes have been proposed: oral-oral, gastric-oral, and fecal-oral.

There has been increasing interest in Hp infection in the oral cavity since the oral-oral route is one of the primary transmission ways. Early diagnosis is essential for treating and controlling Hp infection worldwide.

Besides the role of Hp in the oral cavity has been investigated and studied for the last 30 years, the results obtained to date are antagonistic, perhaps due to the various researchers' different diagnostic methods, the study designs, the inclusion/exclusion criteria, and the selected controls. On the one hand, in patients with BHH in the oral cavity, the dental plaque and lingual dorsum have been identified as Hp reservoirs for colonization. On the other hand, the mouth was also investigated in patients with aphthous stomatitis, cancer, and Sjögren's syndrome [3].

2. Dental plaque and saliva in periodontal disease

Dental plaque, or oral biofilm, is a translucent film that is a mixture of biotic matrix (bacteria, fungi) and intra/extracellular matrix (organic and mineral compounds), which was firmly adhered to tooth surfaces, gingival and oral epithelium, prostheses, and restorations. It is not removable with a simple rinse, and its composition varies depending on the location and maturation time. It is the direct cause of caries and periodontal disease on dental and periodontal surfaces. Dental plaque hosts various bacteria, and in the absence of good oral hygiene, it forms quickly and adheres to the surface of the teeth at the supragingival and subgingival levels.

In 1989, Kradjen and collaborators were the first to isolate Hp by culture from dental plaque in patients with Hp-positive gastric pathology in Canada, but they only found Hp in 1.4% (1/71) cases [4]. In 2001, 108 patients with gastric pathology and Hp-positive dental plaque were identified in Turkey, whose patients with good oral hygiene did not experience reoccurrences after being treated with antibiotic therapy [5]. In Iran, similarities were found between Hp strains isolated from saliva, feces, and gastric samples, indicating the possible role of saliva as a source of Hp infection. However, the diversity of Hp genotypes among the stomach, feces, and saliva in the same patient suggests that more than one Hp strain may exist in the saliva and stomach of the same patient due to coinfection or genetic variation [6]. In global studies, dental plaque has been identified as a reservoir of Hp in the oral cavity and as the gateway for bacteria entering the gastrointestinal system [7]. Proof of this was the clinical trial carried out in the gastroenterology unit of the Sisli Hamidiye Etfal Hospital in Turkey, where Hp was detected in the dental biofilm and saliva of children with gastric Hp, which allowed us to understand that both gastric reinfection and treatment failure could be due to the presence of Hp in the oral cavity [8]. In periodontal lesions, the number of bacteria increases with the development of periodontitis. Along with *Porphyromonas gingivalis* strains, *Fusobacterium nucleatum*, *Fusobacterium periodontium*, and different Hp strains have been found to co-aggregate. The first studies reporting results about the presence of Hp in subgingival plaque from patients with periodontitis were conducted in Finland and Great Britain, with subgingival plaque samples from patients with periodontal disease [9, 10]. The former reported negative results in 100% of patients, while the latter described a Hp positivity of 38% (11/29). Neither researcher assessed gastric conditions [9, 10]. In the third National Health and Nutritional Examination Survey (NHANES III; 1988–1991), 4504 subjects who had undergone anti-Hp therapy and had positive Hp serology were eligible and underwent periodontal evaluation. The results showed that 2% of the population had periodontal disease, with a pocket greater than or equal to 5 mm, with an OR of 1.46 (CI 1.11–1.92), suggesting that periodontitis could be a risk factor for Hp infection [11]. Other researchers have estimated a 60% prevalence of Hp subgingival plaque colonization in patients with gastric involvement, identified by culture and polymerase chain reaction (PCR), reporting a PCR sensitivity of 100% and a specificity of 70% [11]. Systematic reviews and meta-analyses have evaluated the association between periodontal disease and Hp infection in the oral cavity in patients with gastric disease. A 63% reduction in relative risk was observed, concluding that eradication therapy alone does not effectively control gastric reinfection [12–14].

The high prevalence of Hp in dental plaque has shown that the oral cavity can be an essential reservoir of Hp. Poor oral hygiene can lead to reinfection after eradication treatment. Good oral hygiene could contribute positively to the treatment of gastritis. Therefore, oral hygiene education should be provided to patients. More studies are needed to clarify the importance of oral Hp and its relationship with salivary parameters and oral hygiene status [15].

3. Other associated oral pathologies

3.1 Aphthous stomatitis

Aphthous stomatitis is characterized by erosions/ulcerations with a necrotic background, erythematous halo, and an oval shape involving mucous membranes. Its most frequent locations include the labial mucosa, buccal mucosa, mouth floor, tongue's ventral surface, soft palate, tonsillar pillars, and alveolar gingiva [16]. Due to histological similarities with gastric ulcers, an association between Hp and recurrent aphthous stomatitis (RAS) is suggested. However, some studies using serological tests and biopsies failed to show such an association [17, 18]. On the other hand, attempts were also made to establish the role of Hp in the pathogenesis of RAS in patients with HIV, but the results were negative [19]. In addition, the association could not be demonstrated using molecular biology as a diagnostic method [20–25].

The impact of Hp eradication on the clinical course of RAS was investigated in patients with Hp-positive gastric biopsies. It was observed that eradicating Hp significantly increased vitamin B12 levels and reduced the number of lesions in these patients. These facts could be explained by the hypothesis that Hp could potentially multiply in macrophages, dendritic cells, and epithelial cells and then indirectly lead to vitamin B deficiency, which would then cause changes in the epithelium of the tongue and buccal mucosa that would lead to mucosal bleeding and glossitis, given its essential role in DNA synthesis [26, 27].

3.2 Oral cancer

3.2.1 Oral squamous cell carcinoma

Oral squamous cell carcinoma (OSCC) constitutes 90% of oral cancer cases. Risk factors for OSCC include tobacco use, alcohol consumption, and human papillomavirus (HPV) infection, which may modify the oral cavity's microbial composition. The oral microbiota and known OSCC risk factors appear to drive oral carcinogenesis. For instance, oral bacteria can transform alcohol into acetaldehyde, promoting mutagenesis in the oral mucosa [28].

The association between oral cancer and Hp action was hardly investigated in biopsies, swabs, and serum samples searching the bacteria, using culture, serology, histopathology, urease test, CLO test (Campylobacter-like organism test), rapid urease test, and PCR methods [29, 30]. Recent pilot studies have suggested a possible association between Hp and OSCC, but additional research in larger populations is needed to confirm and precisely quantify this potential association [31, 32].

3.2.2 Mucosa-associated lymphoid tissue (MALT) lymphoma

Isaacson and Wright, in 1983, introduced the term mucosa-associated lymphoid tissue (MALT) lymphoma, defined by the WHO as extranodal B-cell lymphoma of the marginal zone of mucosa-associated lymphoid tissue, that represented 10% of all lymphomas and 3% of gastric neoplasms. MALT lymphoma is commonly located at the gastrointestinal level [33, 34]. The causal relationship between Hp infection and gastric MALT lymphoma is supported by its high remission rate after infection resolution (>75%) [35]. Some studies have reported cases in major (parotid) and minor (labial) salivary glands in patients with Sjögren's syndrome associated with Hp infection. Antibiotic therapy contributed to successful Hp eradication and MALT lymphoma resolution [36–38].

3.3 Burning, halitosis, and lingual papillary hypertrophy (BHH)

Halitosis refers to the abnormal odor of exhaled air from the mouth. The term derives from the Latin "halitus" (breath) and the Greek "osis" (disease) [39]. The three main diagnostic methods for halitosis are gas chromatography, organoleptic measurement, and sulfur monitoring [40]. Halitosis has been attributed to various factors, with highlighted gastric imbalances [41].

After Hp eradication therapy in patients with gastric pathology, halitosis disappeared with antibiotic treatment. It was associated with gastric-level Hp infection [42–45]. Researchers suggested that halitosis could be an effective biomarker for predicting erosive changes beyond inflammation in the gastric mucosa of affected patients [46].

Oral halitosis is caused by volatile sulfur compounds (VSCs) generated by bacterial metabolism degrading sulfur in amino acids [47]. Anaerobic and predominantly gram-negative bacteria, found in the gingival sulcus, periodontal pockets, and posterior lingual dorsum, play a crucial role [48]. *Treponema denticola*, *Porphyromonas gingivalis*, *Prevotella intermedia*, *Bacteroides forsythus*, *Fusobacterium periodonticum*, *Centipeda periodontii*, *Porphyromonas endodontalis*, *Fusobacterium nucleatum*, *Veillonella parvula*, *Actinomyces odontolyticus*, *Streptococcus intermedius*, and *Clostridium innocuum* are commonly diagnosed on the dorsum of the tongue [49–51]. Candida, a yeast colonizing the dorsum of the tongue, contains Hp-specific genes. This may explain Hp's presence in the oral cavity, where the environment is adverse. Hp resides within Candida's vacuoles, providing protection [52]. Hp presence was reported in the posterior sector of the lingual dorsum through biopsy with positive PCR results [53].

Patients with BHH may present with both tongue and gastric Hp infections. These patients did not respond effectively to treatment and were diagnosed with chronic candidiasis concerning lingual papillary hypertrophy. They were referred to Periodontics services for Halitosis. A considerable percentage (60%) of these patients had a history of chronic untreated gastric discomfort. Diagnosing Hp in the oral cavity must be confirmed with molecular biology, and the patient's gastric involvement must be evaluated [54, 55].

4. Diagnosis of oral infection by *Helicobacter pylori* (Hp)

Some methods for diagnosing oral Hp infection analyze this bacteria's structural and functional characteristics. Other methods evaluate the immune response it provokes in the host. Not all methods used in the stomach work in the same way. The reasons for choosing one or another diagnostic tool are based on the clinical case and the availability of these methodologies. Any of the methods used to detect Hp in the mouth requires that the patient is not under medication, both oral and general, in the last 4 weeks with simethicone, proton pump inhibitors, histamine H2 blockers, bismuth, antibiotics, antifungals, and mouthwashes. The methods can be invasive, generally based on the study of the biopsy, and non-invasive by studying samples obtained by swab, cytobrush, saliva, or blood.

4.1 Histology

The histological study of the biopsy allows us to identify the oral mucosa lesions but does not detect Hp infection. In 2001, Adler and collaborators identified the Hp genome for the first time in the biopsy of a 35-year-old male patient with halitosis and burning mouth, accompanied by dyspepsia, who at the time of consultation presented hyperplasia of posterior filiform papillae with negative mycological culture and biopsy with active chronic gastritis due to Hp. A partial biopsy of the affected lingual area was performed for histopathological study and determination of Hp by PCR (see Section 5.4). The histopathological study showed marked epithelial hyperplasia, papillomatosis, acanthosis, and hyperparakeratosis. The underlying chorion presented an inflammatory infiltrate composed predominantly of lymphocytes and attached to the surface of the epithelium; there was a thick bacterial plaque with abundant coccoid elements. With the Giemsa technique, spiral bacteria adhered to the epithelial surface were identified, with morphology similar to that of Hp classically described in gastric biopsies (**Figure 1**). Identification of microorganisms by this method requires confirmatory genomic evaluation (see Section 5.2) [56].

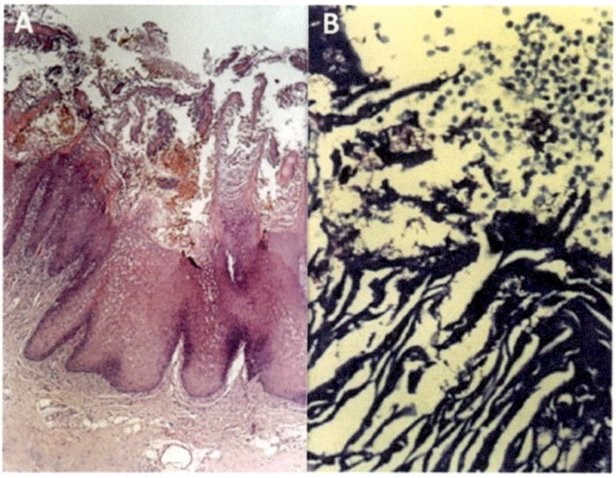

Figure 1.
(A) Epithelial hyperplasia, papillomatosis, acanthosis, and hyperparakeratosis are observed. In the underlying chorion, an inflammatory infiltrate is composed predominantly of lymphocytes. Attached to the surface of the epithelium was a bacterial plaque with abundant coccoid elements (hematoxylin-eosin - HE). (B) Spiral bacteria adhering to the epithelial surface are individualized. The morphology of these elements is similar to that of the Hp described in gastric biopsies (Giemsa) [56].

4.2 Culture

The culture of Hp is a specific method whose sensitivity depends on variables such as sample collection, transportation, storage, culture media used, and incubation conditions (percentage of CO_2 and humidity). Once the sample is obtained, it must be placed in a carbonated Stuart transport medium. This method allows for determining sensitivity to antimicrobials, characterizing virulence factors, and typing strains for epidemiological purposes. This technique is inappropriate in dental plaque and the lingual dorsum due to the presence of coccoid forms of Hp and abundant other accompanying pathogens [57].

4.3 Rapid urease test (RUT)

The rapid urease test is a qualitative test used to detect the presence of Hp by measuring the activity of the bacteria's urease enzyme. The sample is placed in a urea tube containing a pH indicator. Despite being a rapid method for identifying Hp, it would not be specific in the oral cavity because other bacteria have urease activity [58].

4.4 Serological tests

Hp provokes a local and systemic immune response. Serological tests are based on detecting specific circulating antibodies in response to bacterial antigens in saliva or serum. Several serological methods have been developed for detecting Hp, such as bacterial agglutination, complement fixation, indirect immunofluorescence, and enzyme immunoassay techniques. The most used approach is enzyme immunoassay (EIA) and enzyme-linked immunosorbent assay (ELISA) because it is quantitative, allowing treatment monitoring. However, its value in diagnosing Hp infection in the mouth must be interpreted cautiously since a positive result does not determine the ubiquity of Hp. Another local option is to study antibodies in saliva, which is an easy sample to obtain, but the main disadvantage is the low concentration of antibodies in them [59].

4.5 Breath test (urea breath test—UBT)

The breath test or exhaled air test is a non-invasive indirect method. It is based on detecting the presence of Hp urease by taking samples of the patient's breath with C13 (non-radioactive), the first in a basal state and the second 30 minutes after ingesting a solution with urea isotopically labeled or only one sample with C14 (radioactive). If Hp is in the mouth and/or stomach, it hydrolyzes urea thanks to its urease, and labeled CO_2 (C13 or C14) is released, absorbed, diffused into the blood, and released with the breath. A non-radioactive method has similar sensitivity but requires a mass spectrometer to measure. The breath test indicates an active infection because urease is produced in the viable organism. However, its value in diagnosing Hp infection in the mouth must be interpreted cautiously since a positive result does not determine the ubiquity of Hp, and the breath test must not ever be used for oral HP diagnosis due to the presence of other urease-positive microbes [59].

5. Molecular pathology of *Helicobacter pylori* (Hp)

Hp has a small 1.6-Mbp genome compared to many other pathogenic bacteria, consisting of a single circular chromosome that encodes about 1600 proteins.

The Hp core genome consists of approximately 1100 genes. The Hp genome is different between strains and even within the bacteria present in an individual's stomach, resulting from the unusual combination of very high rates of mutation and recombination. This high frequency of mutations can be explained by the lack of proofreading function in the DNA polymerase in combination with the pro-mutagenic properties of its DNA. The diversity of DNA sequences can spread rapidly through Hp populations due to recombination between strains. Hp can be updated extracellularly because its DNA can be recombined, allowing HP to adapt its genome to new environments exceptionally efficiently [60].

5.1 Molecular technique

5.1.1 Polymerase chain reaction (PCR)

Kary B. Mullis obtained The Nobel Prize in Chemistry in 1993 for inventing the PCR process, in which a small amount of DNA can be copied in large quantities over a short period. PCR is based on synthesizing new DNA strands complementary to the template strand present using DNA polymerase that can add a nucleotide to a pre-existing 3′-OH group that will be offered by a primer with complementary sequence to the region of interest that will be mandatorily necessary to add the first nucleotide. Two primers flanking the sequence of interest are needed so that at the end of the PCR reaction, the particular sequence accumulates into billions of copies (amplicons) since the PCR reaction generates copies of the target sequence exponentially (**Figure 2**) [61, 62].

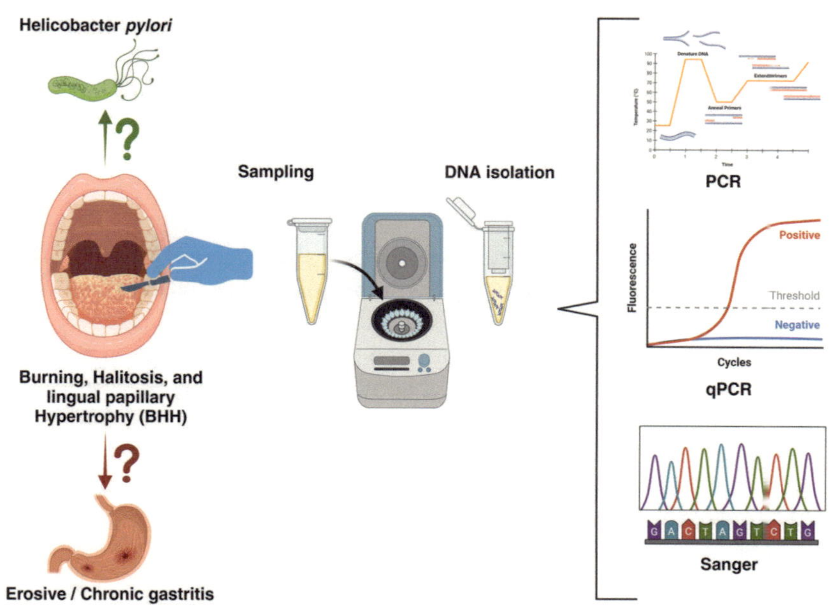

Figure 2.
Halitosis is an effective sign for early diagnosis of Helicobacter pylori *infection, which should be confirmed by molecular techniques and correlated with gastric involvement (Created with BioRender.com).*

5.1.2 Real-time quantitative PCR (qPCR) assays

During the PCR reaction, if one wants to know the initial amount of the target sequence contained in the sample, one must measure the amplification in the exponential phase of the PCR because only in that phase is there a linear relationship between reactive and product. Like any enzymatic reaction, the target sequence ceases to amplify due to the product accumulation, and a "plateau effect" appears. At this point, the endpoint PCR is measured because it is the maximum concentration point of amplicons that the reaction can obtain. This attribute of PCR makes real-time quantitative PCR (qPCR) necessary, which amplifies a targeted DNA molecule during the PCR process (**Figure 2**). There exist at least two methods for detecting PCR products: non-specific fluorescent dyes that bind double-stranded DNA molecules by intercalating between the DNA bases and sequence-specific fluorescence resonance energy transfer probes that only see the amplicon hybridized with its complementary sequence (TaqMan) [63].

5.1.3 Sanger capillary sequencing

Sanger sequencing was first developed by Frederick Sanger and colleagues in 1977 and has become the most widely used sequencing method for over 40 years. It is a DNA sequencing method based on the selective incorporation of chain-terminating dideoxynucleotides (ddNTPs) by DNA polymerase during in vitro DNA replication [63]. DNA polymerase enzyme adds a nucleotide to a pre-existing 3′-OH group of the primer, either deoxynucleotide triphosphates (dNTPs: dATP, dGTP, dCTP, dTTP) or chain-terminating dideoxynucleotide triphosphates (ddNTPs: ddATP, ddGTP, ddCTP, ddTTP) in rate-limiting concentrations which stop the elongation reaction as the ddNTPs are incorporated, resulting in distinguishable DNA fragments of various lengths. A high-quality DNA template is mandatory for sequence analysis. Therefore, storage duration, temperature, and fixatives have an essential impact on the recovery [64]. Sequencing procedures require DNA or RNA amplicons that are longer than those used for qPCR (150 bp) for optimal results (**Figure 2**). Sanger method remains widely used for smaller-scale projects and validation of next-generation sequencing (NGS).

5.1.4 Next-generation sequencing (NGS)

Large-scale parallel sequencing (next-generation sequencing, NGS) is a DNA sequencing technology revolutionizing genomic amplification. NGS can sequence the whole human genome within a single day. Over the last few years, massively parallel sequencing has rapidly evolved and transitioned into molecular pathology routine laboratories. This is an exciting platform for simultaneously analyzing multiple genes with low input material. The spectrum of DNA variation in a human genome comprises small base changes (substitutions), insertions and deletions of DNA, large genomic deletions of exons or whole genes, and rearrangements, such as inversions and translocations [63]. This methodology could be used to analyze Hp resistance in an automated way, as well as the classification of bacterial strains.

5.2 Tissue sampling

The central dogma of molecular biology explains the flow of genetic information within a biological system: "DNA makes RNA, and RNA makes protein," the analysis of each biomolecule is called genomics, transcriptomics, and proteomics, respectively. This chapter focused on a Hp genomic approach, and it should be emphasized that genomic research is an indirect viability measure because it does not imply an active bacterial infection. Therefore, a genomic approach performed from fresh frozen tissue (FFT) complements the clinical lesion observed, and served from formalin-fixed paraffin-embedded tissue (FFPET) complements the histological characteristics.

5.2.1 Fresh frozen tissue (FFT)

Fresh frozen tissue (FFT) is the "gold standard" type of biosample for PCR and especially for sequencing. However, frozen tissue collection is generally not feasible because clinical workflows provide formalin-fixed material that, unfortunately, allows less DNA to be obtained, which is usually more degraded than in fresh samples, which produces sequencing artifacts associated with the fixation process [64].

5.2.2 Formalin-fixed paraffin-embedded tissue (FFPET)

Formalin-fixed, paraffin-embedded tissue (FFEPT) block is the "gold standard" method of human tissue preservation for diagnosis. The fixation of tissue specimens by formalin has been used for almost 120 years. A formalin concentration of 10% was suggested, which is equivalent to a final formaldehyde concentration of 4% [65]. Processing samples in this manner has several advantages; on the one hand, it mitigates risks of infectious agents that may be present in the fresh material. On the other hand, it ensures the preservation of the architectural components of the tissue, and it allows, through thin sections, to examine the architecture of the tissue using simple dyes, such as hematoxylin and eosin [66].

Fixation damages the structure of DNA and thus negatively affects subsequent PCR. For example, tissues fixed for 8 days can amplify 536-bp fragments, and for 30 days, only 268-bp [67]. Due to this fragmentation, quantification before performing a molecular technique was mandatory. Quantification and purity evaluation of nucleic acids are generally performed by spectrophotometric analysis or ultraviolet fluorescence tagging. Ultraviolet wavelength light (260 nm) absorption is directly related to the sample's nucleic acid concentration. Purity assessments are employed to detect (i) contaminating proteins with a peak absorption of 280 nm, particularly from the aromatic amino acids, with a sample's 260 nm/280 nm absorbance ratio > 1.8 ratio; (ii) other contaminants with a peak absorption on 230 nm, particularly from carbohydrates, phenol, guanidine, and glycogen, with a sample's 260 nm/230 nm absorbance ratio of 2.0–2.2 [64].

5.3 PCR amplicon size

Ideal amplicon length/size depends on many variables and design preferences. For standard PCR, scientists generally design amplicons between 200 and 1000 bp. However, for quantitative PCR, expected amplicons range from 75 to 150 bp. But, as mentioned above, fixation breaks the genetic material, and PCR performed in FFPET needs a design of specific-sequence primers that flank targets with molecular weights less than 300 bp.

There are different genetic targets of Hp. The most used target gene in the literature was the 16S rRNA, but they also used cagA, vacA genes, and urease A [3]. The selection depends on the amplified fragment's sensitivity and specificity according

	FFT	FFPET
End point PCR	200–1000	<300 bp
Quantitative PCR	<150 bp	
Sanger sequencing	>150 bp	>150 bp

Table 1.
Amplicon size concerning sample type and molecular biology methods (FFT: fresh frozen tissue, FFPET: formalin-fixed paraffin-embedded tissue).

to the primers' design that defines a specific size, allowing different amplification methods depending on the patient's sample (**Table 1**).

5.4 *Helicobacter pylori* molecular approach

Based on the test, laboratory equipment available, and the patient clinical characteristics, the optimal diagnostic approach requires weighing several factors.

As mentioned above, Adler et al. described a case report in 2001 that, for the first time, identified Hp in BHH. The FFPET biopsy was histologically analyzed with HE and Giemsa staining, while Hp DNA was detected by PCR [56]. The primers used for gastric biopsies in FFPET were employed in this first oral case. The Hp genome was studied with a semiquantitative molecular technique (PCR), with primers homologous to a region that codes for the species-specific antigen. Their nucleotide sequence was HP3: 5′-TGGCGTGTCTATTGACAGCGAGC-3′ and HP4: 5′-CCTGCTGGGCATACTTCACCATG-3′, identified with 474–496 and 776–754 residue peptides, respectively, that flank a 298-bp amplicon [68]. Negative, positive, and blank controls were used. On the other hand, a second PCR was carried out under similar conditions for a 110 bp region of the human beta-globin gene, as amplification control of a DNA patient using the oligonucleotide primers PC03 and PC04 [69]. All these PCRs were analyzed with 9% polyacrylamide gel electrophoresis in TBE 1X buffer (Tris-Boric-EDTA) and visualized with ethidium bromide under ultraviolet light. As the fragment was more significant than 150 bp (**Table 1**), two-way Sanger sequencing could be performed and aligned by basic local alignment search tool (BLAST) with the Hp genome. By 2005, Adler et al. increased the study population. They studied extensively patients with BHH by molecular methods, intending to confirm the relationship between BHH and Hp reliably [54]. DNA was purified from 7-μm sections of the lingual mucosa biopsies of the affected site, which were formalin-fixed paraffin-embedded. The same protocol as in 2001 was followed. Still, the positive results of Hp were confirmed with a second PCR, with sequence-specific primers that amplified a 109 bp region of the 16Sr RNA gene HP1: 5′-CTGGAGAGACTAAGCCCTCC-3′ and HP2: 5′-ATTACTGACGCTGATTGTGC-3′ [70]. This study of two different genomic targets confirmed the linkage of BHH with the presence of the Hp genome.

By 2014, Adler's group decided to convert the method to a less invasive test by sampling the lingual dorsum by scraping and performing PCR from fresh tissue to increase sensitivity, specificity, and speed of results [3]. For this purpose, primers were used to allow qualitative end-point PCR assays but with the possibility of using the same design in a real-time PCR. The primer that amplifies a 114-bp fragment corresponding to the 16S rRNA gene of Hp was 16S2-F:5′-CGCTAAGAGATCAGCCTATGTCC-3′ and 16SB2-R: 5′-CCGTGTTCTCAGTTCCAGTGTGT-3′ (GenBank: U00679.1) [71]. Quantifying the bacterial inoculum allows clinical monitoring of patients and evaluation of the response to local treatment. However, quantitative methods should be performed on fresh samples.

6. Treatment with effectiveness in the oral cavity

Before the discovery of Hp in the 1980s, peptic ulcer was considered a chronic disease: "Once there is an ulcer, there is always an ulcer," but once the bacterial infection was described as the cause of the pathogen, it was transformed into a unique disease, since healing Hp infection prevents ulcer recurrence and the development of new peptic ulcers. Despite the recognition that Hp is the leading cause of atrophic gastritis, the hypothesis that its eradication could prevent and reduce the incidence of gastric cancer was slowly accepted. More than a decade passed after Hp was defined as a human carcinogen for acceptance that curing the infection also reduces the incidence and prevents the development of gastric cancer [72].

Effective Hp therapy may include an antisecretory drug, antimicrobials to reduce the chances of survival of pre-existing resistant subpopulations, and bismuth. The most used therapy is the 14-day triple therapy consisting of a combination of three drugs, a proton pump inhibitor (PPI), and two antibiotics, which can be amoxicillin and clarithromycin, one of which can be replaced in particular cases by metronidazole. Other options are quadruple therapy with bismuth, triple therapies with levofloxacin, or 7-day triple therapies with vonoprazan. Resistance to these combinations has been described, resulting in a lower effectiveness rate [73, 74]. After successful treatment, the oral cavity is a reservoir for gastric re-infection [75]. In Korea, applying a general eradication regimen with red ginseng supplementation at the local level showed eradication rates of 93% [76]. Adler's group, based on the case report of a male patient with Hp infection, both in the mouth (BHH) and in the stomach, established triple therapy in their patients at a general level and added oral hygiene teaching, periodontal treatment, cleaning the tongue with a gauze soaked with mouthwash and topical application of metronidazole gel on the dorsum of the tongue, with a decrease in the recurrence rate of Hp after eradication [56, 77, 78]. The literature on clarithromycin's effects on the lingual surface is old and scarce, and studies that address this treatment in this organ are needed. Still, the use of systemic antibiotics, such as clarithromycin, has been reported to be associated with adverse effects in the oral cavity, such as glossitis that exacerbates BHH syndrome (**Figure 3**) [79].

The diagnosis of candidiasis should be made by mycological culture and fungigram to confirm the species which co-infected the lesion (*Candida albicans*, *dubliniensis*, *kefir*, etc.) and indicate a precise treatment against the species found associated with the information on its therapeutic sensitivity (**Figure 4**).

Infection control includes preventive environmental and oral hygiene measures and regular dental and gastroenterological consultations. Good oral hygiene could contribute positively to the treatment of gastritis. Therefore, oral hygiene education should be provided to patients. More studies are needed to clarify the importance of oral Hp and its relationship with salivary parameters and oral hygiene status [15]. It has been shown that the prevalence of Hp is 20% in urban areas. Still, in rural areas, it exceeds 60%, suggesting that sociocultural and economic factors could determine these differences because they reflect different levels of hygiene, sanitation, living density, and education [78]. However, BHH syndrome does not improve only with good hygiene; it is necessary to administer additional local pharmacological therapy and have periodic consultations with the specialist.

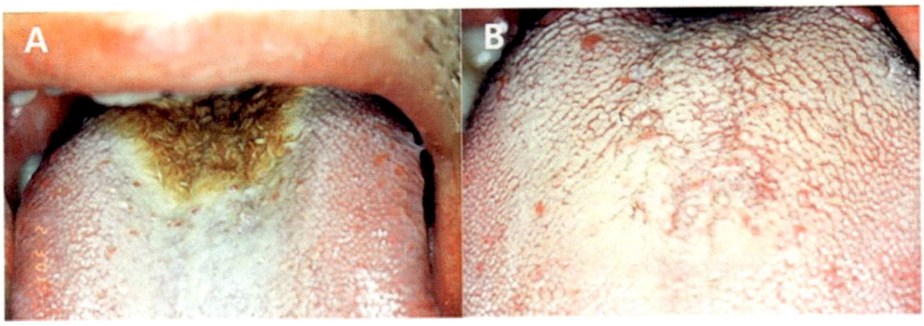

Figure 3.
(A) Patient with BHH and Hp-positive gastritis, confirmed by PCR technique. (B) Post triple therapy and local medication in the tongue. The evolution of BHH was observed after 7 days [56].

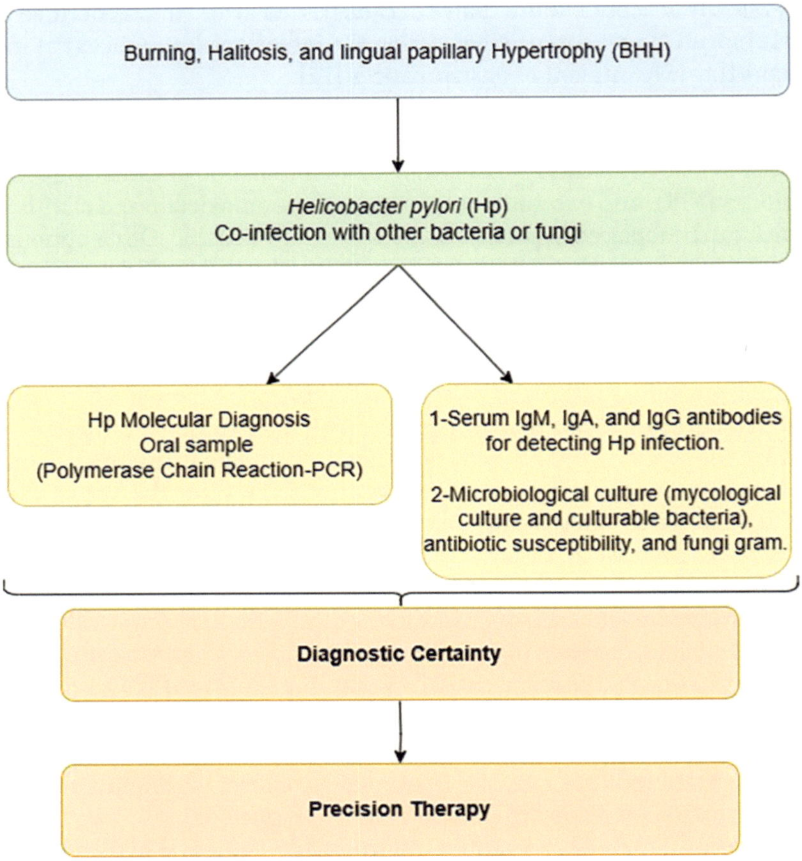

Figure 4.
Diagnosis and treatment algorism of Helicobacter pylori *(Hp) oral infection.*

7. *Helicobacter pylori* challenges

Hp infection, which affects approximately half of the world's population, remains a severe public health problem. Li et al. identified a lower prevalence of Hp infection in younger people, high-income countries, or countries with high levels of universal health coverage. Studies based on serological diagnostic methods generally reported higher Hp prevalence than studies based on non-serological methods (53% vs. 41%) [80]. Hp leads to several gastric pathologies, including inflammation, gastroduodenal ulcers, and malignancies. Early detection and treatment are crucial to preventing the spread of the infection [81].

Precision medicine is an innovative approach to disease prevention and treatment that considers differences in people's genes, injuries, environments, and lifestyles to target the right therapies to the right patients at the right time [82]. In this new approach to Hp infection medicine, the challenges could be:

- To identify germline pathogenic variants in homologous-recombination genes (ATM, BRCA1, BRCA2, CDH1, MLH1, MSH2, MSH6, and PALB2) by NGS, considering that individuals with Hp infection and this germline altered genes had a higher cumulative risk of gastric cancer than non-carriers infected with Hp (45% vs. 14%) [83].

- To confirm if Hp reduces treatment efficacy with immune checkpoint inhibitors in malignant diseases before developing a vaccine for preventive and therapeutic purposes that might consider multiple epitopes to direct the immune response toward essential Hp functions such as epithelial cell adherence, proliferation, and survival in the specific gastric niche [60].

- To incorporate nanoparticles and microparticles in clinical trials to overcome the barriers of the oral route, physicochemical inconveniences, and lack of selectivity of current therapy. Standard oral treatment fails in 20% of cases since the obstacles of the oral route decrease the bioavailability of antibiotics, increasing the rates of resistance [84].

- To develop a new treatment against the redox switch protein HP1021, which controls the transcription of 497 genes, including 407 genes related to response to oxidative stress, that allow Hp to combat stress factors, including reactive oxygen species (ROS) [85].

8. Conclusions

Hp infection is one of the most common infections in the world, and early diagnosis and treatment are essential for its control. One of the strategies for early diagnosis is to detect Hp in BHH, especially in patients with gastric pathologies. The diagnostic method of choice for Hp infection in the mouth is genome detection by PCR. Infection control consists of preventive environmental and oral hygiene measures and regular dental and gastroenterological consultations. Therapeutic measures should consider the joint treatment of oral and gastric pathology, trying in the future to approach precision medicine with massive genetic analysis of the resistance to treatments that the bacterium acquires rapidly due to its high mutation rate, as well as the possible identification of germline variants of the host that increase the risk of gastric cancer in patients already infected.

Acknowledgements

We thank Drs. Elsner, Avagnina, and Fresno for their unconditional support, as well as the staff and patients of the Stomatological Clinic of the University of Buenos Aires (UBA).

Conflict of interest

The authors declare no conflict of interest.

Author details

Isabel Adler[1], Andrea Muiño[1*], Pablo Rodríguez[2] and Valeria Denninghoff[3,4*]

1 Stomatology, Faculty of Dentistry, University of Buenos Aires (UBA), Buenos Aires, Argentina

2 Endodontology, Faculty of Dentistry, University of Buenos Aires (UBA), Buenos Aires, Argentina

3 Molecular Clinical Lab, University of Buenos Aires (UBA) - National Scientific and Technical Research Council (CONICET), Buenos Aires, Argentina

4 Liquid Biopsy and Cancer Interception Unit, GENYO, Centre for Genomics and Oncological Research (Pfizer/University of Granada/Andalusian Regional Government), Granada, Spain

*Address all correspondence to: andrea.muino@odontologia.uba.ar and vdenninghoff@conicet.gov.ar

References

[1] Marshall BJ, Warren JR. Unidentified curved bacilli in the stomach of patients with gastritis and peptic ulceration. Lancet. 1984;**1**:1311-1135. DOI: 10.1016/s0140-6736(84)91816-6

[2] Yee JK. *Helicobacter pylori* colonization of the oral cavity: A milestone discovery. World Journal of Gastroenterology. 2016;**22**:641-648. DOI: 10.3748/wjg.v22.i2.641

[3] Adler I, Muiño A, Aguas S, Harada L, Diaz M, Lence A, et al. *Helicobacter pylori* and oral pathology: Relationship with the gastric infection. World Journal of Gastroenterology. 2014;**20**:9922-9935. DOI: 10.3748/wjg.v20.i29.9922

[4] Krajden S, Fuksa M, Anderson J, Kempston J, Boccia A, Petrea C, et al. Examination of human stomach biopsies, saliva, and dental plaque for *Campylobacter pylori*. Journal of Clinical Microbiology. 1989;**27**:1397-1398. DOI: 10.1128/jcm.27.6.1397-1398.1989

[5] Avcu N, Avcu F, Beyan C, Ural AU, Kaptan K, Ozyurt M, et al. The relationship between gastric-oral *Helicobacter pylori* and oral hygiene in patients with vitamin B12-deficiency anemia. Oral Surgery, Oral Medicine, Oral Pathology, Oral Radiology, and Endodontics. 2001;**92**:166-169. DOI: 10.1067/moe.2001.113589

[6] Momtaz H, Souod N, Dabiri H, Sarshar M. Study of *Helicobacter pylori* genotype status in saliva, dental plaques, stool and gastric biopsy samples. World Journal of Gastroenterology. 2012;**18**:2105-2111. DOI: 10.3748/wjg.v18.i17.2105

[7] Wang XM, Yee KC, Hazeki-Taylor N, Li J, Fu HY, Huang ML, et al. Oral *Helicobacter pylori*, its relationship to successful eradication of gastric *H. pylori* and saliva culture confirmation. Journal of Physiology and Pharmacology. 2014;**65**:559-566

[8] Aksit Bıcak D, Akyuz S, Kıratlı B, Usta M, Urganci N, Alev B, et al. The investigation of *Helicobacter pylori* in the dental biofilm and saliva samples of children with dyspeptic complaints. BMC Oral Health. 2017;**17**:67-78. DOI: 10.1186/s12903-017-0361-x

[9] Asikainen S, Chen C, Slots J. Absence of *Helicobacter pylori* in subgingival samples determined by polymerase chain reaction. Oral Microbiology and Immunology. 1994;**9**:318-320. DOI: 10.1111/j.1399-302x.1994.tb00079.x

[10] Dye BA, Kruszon-Moran D, McQuillan G. The relationship between periodontal disease attributes and *Helicobacter pylori* infection among adults in the United States. American Journal of Public Health. 2002;**92**:1809-1815. DOI: 10.2105/ajph.92.11.1809

[11] Agarwal S, Jithendra KD. Presence of *Helicobacter pylori* in subgingival plaque of periodontitis patients with and without dyspepsia, detected by polymerase chain reaction and culture. Journal of Indian Society of Periodontology. 2012;**16**:398-403. DOI: 10.4103/0972-124X.100919

[12] Bouziane A, Ahid S, Abouqal R, Ennibi O. Effect of periodontal therapy on prevention of gastric *Helicobacter pylori* recurrence: A systematic review and meta-analysis. Journal of Clinical Periodontology. 2012;**39**:1165-1173. DOI: 10.1111/jcpe.12015

[13] Liu Y, Li R, Xue X, Xu T, Luo Y, Dong Q, et al. Periodontal disease and

Helicobacter pylori infection in oral cavity: A meta-analysis of 2727 participants mainly based on Asian studies. Clinical Oral Investigations. 2020l;**24**:2175-2188. DOI: 10.1007/s00784-020-03330-4

[14] Dane A, Gurbuz T. Clinical comparative study of the effects of *Helicobacter pylori* colonization on oral health in children. Pakistan Journal of Medical Sciences. 2016;**32**:969-973. DOI: 10.12669/pjms.324.10034

[15] Anand PS, Kamath KP, Anil S. Role of dental plaque, saliva and periodontal disease in *Helicobacter pylori* infection. World Journal of Gastroenterology. 2014;**20**:5639-5653. DOI: 10.3748/wjg.v20.i19.5639

[16] Edward W. Odell Cawson's Essentials of Oral Pathology and Oral Medicine. 9th ed. Elsevier Health Sciences; 2017. pp. 253-281. ISBN 9780702049811

[17] Riggio MP, Lennon A, Wray D. Detection of *Helicobacter pylori* DNA in recurrent aphthous stomatitis tissue by PCR. Journal of Oral Pathology & Medicine. 2000;**29**:507-513. DOI: 10.1034/j.1600-0714.2000.291005.x

[18] Porter SR, Barker GR, Scully C, Macfarlane G, Bain L. Serum IgG antibodies to *Helicobacter pylori* in patients with recurrent aphthous stomatitis and other oral disorders. Oral Surgery, Oral Medicine, Oral Pathology, Oral Radiology, and Endodontics. 1997;**83**:325-328. DOI: 10.1016/s1079-2104(97)90237-7

[19] Leimola-Virtanen R, Happonen RP, Syrjänen S. Cytomegalovirus (CMV) and *Helicobacter pylori* (HP) found in oral mucosal ulcers. Journal of Oral Pathology & Medicine. 1995;**24**:14-47. DOI: 10.1111/j.1600-0714.1995.tb01123.x

[20] Birek C, Grandhi R, McNeill K, Singer D, Ficarra G, Bowden G. Detection of *Helicobacter pylori* in oral aphthous ulcers. Journal of Oral Pathology & Medicine. 1999;**28**:197-203. DOI: 10.1111/j.1600-0714.1999.tb02024.x

[21] Victória JM, Kalapothakis E, Silva Jde F, Gomez RS. *Helicobacter pylori* DNA in recurrent aphthous stomatitis. Journal of Oral Pathology & Medicine. 2003;**32**:219-223. DOI: 10.1034/j.1600-0714.2003.00136.x

[22] Iamaroon A, Chaimano S, Linpisarn S, Pongsiriwet S, Phornphutkul K. Detection of *Helicobacter pylori* in recurrent aphthous ulceration by nested PCR. Journal of Oral Science. 2003;**45**:107-110. DOI: 10.2334/josnusd.45.107

[23] Fritscher AM, Cherubini K, Chies J, Dias AC. Association between *Helicobacter pylori* and recurrent aphthous stomatitis in children and adolescents. Journal of Oral Pathology & Medicine. 2004;**33**:129-132. DOI: 10.1111/j.0904-2512.2004.00074.x

[24] Mansour-Ghanaei F, Asmar M, Bagherzadeh AH, Ekbataninezhad S. *Helicobacter pylori* infection in oral lesions of patients with recurrent aphthous stomatitis. Medical Science Monitor. 2005;**11**:576-579

[25] Gomes CC, Gomez RS, Zina LG, Amaral FR. Recurrent aphthous stomatitis and *Helicobacter pylori*. Medicina Oral, Patología Oral y Cirugía Bucal. 2016;**21**:e187-e191. DOI: 10.4317/medoral.20872

[26] Taş DA, Yakar T, Sakalli H, Serin E. Impact of *Helicobacter pylori* on the clinical course of recurrent aphthous stomatitis. Journal of Oral Pathology & Medicine. 2013;**42**:89-94. DOI: 10.1111/j.1600-0714.2012.01197.x

[27] Gao Y, Gupta N, Abdalla M. Recurrent aphthous stomatitis improved after eradication therapy for *Helicobacter pylori*. Case Reports in Gastrointestinal Medicine. 2021;**2021**:5543838. DOI: 10.1155/2021/5543838

[28] Chen J, Domingue JC, Sears CL. Microbiota dysbiosis in select human cancers: Evidence of association and causality. Seminars in Immunology. 2017;**32**:25-34. DOI: 10.1016/j.smim.2017.08.001

[29] Grandis JR, Perez-Perez GI, Yu VL, Johnson JT, Blaser MJ. Lack of serologic evidence for *Helicobacter pylori* infection in head and neck cancer. Head & Neck. 1997;**19**:216-218. DOI: 10.1002/(sici)1097-0347(199705)19:3<216::aid-hed9>3.0.co;2-5

[30] Meng X, Wang Q, He C, Chen M, Liu J, Liu W, et al. An inverse association of *Helicobacter pylori* infection with oral squamous cell carcinoma. Journal of Oral Pathology & Medicine. 2016;**45**:17-22. DOI: 10.1111/jop.12324

[31] Dayama A, Srivastava V, Shukla M, Singh R, Pandey M. *Helicobacter pylori* and oral cancer: Possible association in a preliminary case control study. Asian Pacific Journal of Cancer Prevention. 2011;**12**:1333-1336

[32] Mohtasham N, Saghravanian N, Zare R, Saghafi S, Ghazi N, Mohajertehran F, et al. Tumor tissue *Helicobacter pylori* and human papillomavirus infection in head and neck squamous cell carcinoma patients and association with clinicopathological indices: A cross-sectional medical survey. Dental Research Journal (Isfahan). 2022;**19**:8. DOI: 10.4103/1735-3327.336693

[33] Isaacson P, Wright DH. Malignant lymphoma of mucosa-associated lymphoid tissue. A distinctive type of B-cell lymphoma. Cancer. 1983; **52**:1410-1406. DOI: 10.1002/1097-0142(19831015)52:8<1410::aid-cncr2820520813>3.0.co;2-3

[34] Harris NL, Jaffe ES, Diebold J, Flandrin G, Muller-Hermelink HK, Vardiman J, et al. The World Health Organization classification of neoplasms of the hematopoietic and lymphoid tissues: Report of the Clinical Advisory Committee meeting—Airlie House, Virginia, November, 1997. The Hematology Journal. 2000;**1**:53-66. DOI: 10.1038/sj.thj.6200013

[35] Stolte M, Eidt S. Healing gastric MALT lymphomas by eradicating *H pylori*? Lancet. 1993;**342**:568. DOI: 10.1016/0140-6736(93)91404-a

[36] Nishimura M, Miyajima S, Okada N. Salivary gland MALT lymphoma associated with *Helicobacter pylori* infection in a patient with Sjögren's syndrome. The Journal of Dermatology. 2000;**27**:450-452. DOI: 10.1111/j.1346-8138.2000.tb02204.x

[37] Iwai H, Nakamichi N, Nakae K, Konishi M, Inaba M, Hoshino S, et al. Parotid mucosa-associated lymphoid tissue lymphoma regression after *Helicobacter pylori* eradication. The Laryngoscope. 2009;**119**:1491-1494. DOI: 10.1002/lary.20258

[38] Keszler A, Adler LI, Gandolfo MS, Masquijo Bisio PA, Smith AC, Vollenweider CF, et al. MALT lymphoma in labial salivary gland biopsy from Sjögren syndrome: Importance of follow-up in early detection. Oral Surgery, Oral Medicine, Oral Pathology, Oral Radiology. 2013;**115**:e28-e33. DOI: 10.1016/j.oooo.2012.07.481

[39] Tangerman A. Halitosis in medicine: A review. International Dental Journal. 2002;**52**:201-306. DOI: 10.1002/j.1875-595x.2002.tb00925.x

[40] Yaegaki K, Coil JM. Examination, classification, and treatment of halitosis; clinical perspectives. Journal of the Canadian Dental Association. 2000;**66**:257-261

[41] Delanghe G, Ghyselen J, van Steenberghe D, Feenstra L. Multidisciplinary breath-odour clinic. Lancet. 1997;**350**:187. DOI: 10.1016/S0140-6736(05)62354-9

[42] Tiomny E, Arber N, Moshkowitz M, Peled Y, Gilat T. Halitosis and *Helicobacter pylori*. A possible link? Journal of Clinical Gastroenterology. 1992;**15**:236-237. DOI: 10.1097/00004836-199210000-00013

[43] Ierardi E, Amoruso A, La Notte T, Francavilla R, Castellaneta S, Marrazza E, et al. Halitosis and *Helicobacter pylori*: A possible relationship. Digestive Diseases and Sciences. 1998;**43**:2733-2737. DOI: 10.1023/a:1026619831442

[44] Katsinelos P, Tziomalos K, Chatzimavroudis G, Vasiliadis T, Katsinelos T, Pilpilidis I, et al. Eradication therapy in *Helicobacter pylori*-positive patients with halitosis: Long-term outcome. Medical Principles and Practice. 2007;**16**:119-123. DOI: 10.1159/000098364

[45] Moshkowitz M, Horowitz N, Leshno M, Halpern Z. Halitosis and gastroesophageal reflux disease: A possible association. Oral Diseases. 2007;**13**:581-585. DOI: 10.1111/j.1601-0825.2006.01341.x

[46] Yoo SH, Jung HS, Sohn WS, Kim BH, Ku BH, Kim YS, et al. Volatile sulfur compounds as a predictor for esophagogastroduodenal mucosal injury. Gut and Liver. 2008;**2**:113-118. DOI: 10.5009/gnl.2008.2.2.113

[47] Kazor CE, Mitchell PM, Lee AM, Stokes LN, Loesche WJ, Dewhirst FE, et al. Diversity of bacterial populations on the tongue dorsa of patients with halitosis and healthy patients. Journal of Clinical Microbiology. 2003;**41**:558-563. DOI: 10.1128/JCM.41.2.558-563.2003

[48] Rosenberg M. Clinical assessment of bad breath: Current concepts. Journal of the American Dental Association (1939). 1996;**127**:475-382. DOI: 10.14219/jada.archive.1996.0239

[49] De Boever EH, Loesche WJ. Assessing the contribution of anaerobic microflora of the tongue to oral malodor. Journal of the American Dental Association (1939). 1995;**126**:1384-1393. DOI: 10.14219/jada.archive.1995.0049

[50] Scully C, el-Maaytah M, Porter SR, Greenman J. Breath odor: Etiopathogenesis, assessment and management. European Journal of Oral Sciences. 1997;**105**:287-293. DOI: 10.1111/j.1600-0722.1997.tb00242.x

[51] Riggio MP, Lennon A, Rolph HJ, Hodge PJ, Donaldson A, Maxwell AJ, et al. Molecular identification of bacteria on the tongue dorsum of subjects with and without halitosis. Oral Diseases. 2008;**14**:251-258. DOI: 10.1111/j.1601-0825.2007.01371.x

[52] Siavoshi F, Saniee P. Vacuoles of *Candida* yeast as a specialized niche for *Helicobacter pylori*. World Journal of Gastroenterology. 2014;**20**:5263-5273. DOI: 10.3748/wjg.v20.i18.5263

[53] Gall-Troselj K, Mravak-Stipetić M, Jurak I, Ragland WL, Pavelić J. *Helicobacter pylori* colonization of tongue mucosa—Increased incidence in atrophic glossitis and burning mouth syndrome (BMS). Journal of Oral Pathology & Medicine. 2001;**30**:560-563. DOI: 10.1034/j.1600-0714.2001.300909.x

[54] Adler I, Denninghoff VC, Alvarez MI, Avagnina A, Yoshida R,

Elsner B. *Helicobacter pylori* associated with glossitis and halitosis. Helicobacter. 2005;**10**:312-317. DOI: 10.1111/j.1523-5378.2005.00322.x

[55] Zhao Y, Gao X, Guo J, Yu D, Xiao Y, Wang H, et al. *Helicobacter pylori* infection alters gastric and tongue coating microbial communities. Helicobacter. 2019;**24**:e12567. DOI: 10.1111/hel.12567

[56] Adler I, Denninghoff V, Alvarez MI, Pecollo J, Neffen E, Avagnina A, et al. Infeccion intrabucal por helicobacter en paciente de sexo masculino. Revista del Ateneo Argentino de Odontología. 2001;**40**:10-15

[57] Allaker RP, Young KA, Hardie JM, Domizio P, Meadows NJ. Prevalence of *Helicobacter pylori* at oral and gastrointestinal sites in children: Evidence for possible oral-to-oral transmission. Journal of Medical Microbiology. 2002;**51**:312-317. DOI: 10.1099/0022-1317-51-4-312

[58] McNicholl AG, Ducons J, Barrio J, Bujanda L, Forné-Bardera M, Aparcero R, et al. Accuracy of the ultra-rapid urease test for diagnosis of *Helicobacter pylori* infection. Gastroenterología y Hepatología. 2017;**40**:651-657. DOI: 10.1016/j.gastrohep.2017.07.007

[59] McNulty CA, Wyatt JI. ACP. Best practice no 154. February 1999. *Helicobacter pylori*. Journal of Clinical Pathology. 1999;**52**:338-344. DOI: 10.1136/jcp.52.5.338

[60] Malfertheiner P, Camargo MC, El-Omar E, Liou JM, Peek R, Schulz C, et al. *Helicobacter pylori* infection. Nature Reviews. Disease Primers. 2023;**9**:19. DOI: 10.1038/s41572-023-00431-8

[61] Mullis K, Faloona F, Scharf S, Saiki R, Horn G, Erlich H. Specific enzymatic amplification of DNA in vitro: The polymerase chain reaction. Cold Spring Harbor Symposia on Quantitative Biology. 1986;**51**:263-273. DOI: 10.1101/sqb.1986.051.01.032

[62] Mullis KB. The unusual origin of the polymerase chain reaction. Scientific American. 1990;**262**:56-65. DOI: 10.1038/scientificamerican0490-56

[63] Denninghoff V. Molecular pathology in the new age of personalized medicine. In: Pathology—From Classics to Innovations. London, UK, London, UK: IntechOpen; 2021. DOI: 10.5772/intechopen.94927

[64] Crossley BM, Bai J, Glaser A, Maes R, Porter E, Killian ML, et al. Guidelines for sanger sequencing and molecular assay monitoring. Journal of Veterinary Diagnostic Investigation. 2020;**32**:767-775. DOI: 10.1177/1040638720905833

[65] Lenze D, Müller HH, Hummel M. Considerations for the use of formalin-fixed and paraffin-embedded tissue specimens for clonality analysis. Journal of Hematopathology. 2012;**5**:27-34. DOI: 10.1007/s12308-012-0138-8

[66] Mathieson W, Thomas GA. Why formalin-fixed, paraffin-embedded biospecimens must be used in genomic medicine: An evidence-based review and conclusion. The Journal of Histochemistry and Cytochemistry. 2020;**68**:543-552. DOI: 10.1369/0022155420945050

[67] Greer CE, Lund JK, Manos MM. PCR amplification from paraffin-embedded tissues: Recommendations on fixatives for long-term storage and prospective studies. PCR Methods and Applications. 1991;**1**:46-50. DOI: 10.1101/gr.1.1.46

[68] Hammar M, Tyszkiewicz T, Wadström T, O'Toole PW. Rapid

detection of *Helicobacter pylori* in gastric biopsy material by polymerase chain reaction. Journal of Clinical Microbiology. 1992;**30**:54-58. DOI: 10.1128/jcm.30.1.54-58.1992

[69] Saiki RK, Scharf S, Faloona F, Mullis KB, Horn GT, Erlich HA, et al. Enzymatic amplification of beta-globin genomic sequences and restriction site analysis for diagnosis of sickle cell anemia. Science. 1985;**230**:1350-1354. DOI: 10.1126/science.2999980

[70] Oshowo A, Tunio M, Gillam D, Botha AJ, Holton J, Boulos P, et al. Oral colonization is unlikely to play an important role in *Helicobacter pylori* infection. The British Journal of Surgery. 1998;**85**:850-852. DOI: 10.1046/j.1365-2168.1998.00724.x

[71] Osaki T, Matsuki T, Asahara T, Zaman C, Hanawa T, Yonezawa H, et al. Comparative analysis of gastric bacterial microbiota in Mongolian gerbils after long-term infection with *Helicobacter pylori*. Microbial Pathogenesis. 2012;**53**:12-18. DOI: 10.1016/j.micpath.2012.03.008

[72] Lee YC, Dore MP, Graham DY. Diagnosis and treatment of *Helicobacter pylori* infection. Annual Review of Medicine. 2022;**73**:183-195. DOI: 10.1146/annurev-med-042220-020814

[73] Hu Y, Zhu Y, Lu NH. Novel and effective therapeutic regimens for *Helicobacter pylori* in an era of increasing antibiotic resistance. Frontiers in Cellular and Infection Microbiology. 2017;**7**:168. DOI: 10.3389/fcimb.2017.00168

[74] Dore MP, Lu H, Graham DY. Role of bismuth in improving *Helicobacter pylori* eradication with triple therapy. Gut. 2016;**65**:870-878. DOI: 10.1136/gutjnl-2015-311019

[75] Gisbert JP. The recurrence of *Helicobacter pylori* infection: Incidence and variables influencing it. A critical review. The American Journal of Gastroenterology. 2005;**100**:2083-2099. DOI: 10.1111/j.1572-0241.2005.50043.x

[76] Lee JS, Kwon KA, Jung HS, Kim JH, Hahm KB. Korea red ginseng on *Helicobacter pylori*-induced halitosis: Newer therapeutic strategy and a plausible mechanism. Digestion. 2009;**80**:192-199. DOI: 10.1159/000229997

[77] Zhang L, Chen X, Ren B, Zhou X, Cheng L. *Helicobacter pylori* in the oral cavity: Current evidence and potential survival strategies. International Journal of Molecular Sciences. 2022;**23**:13646. DOI: 10.3390/ijms232113646

[78] Katelaris P, Hunt R, Bazzoli F, Cohen H, Fock KM, Gemilyan M, et al. *Helicobacter pylori* world gastroenterology organization global guideline. Journal of Clinical Gastroenterology. 2023;**57**:111-126. DOI: 0.1097/MCG.0000000000001719

[79] Aziz Y, Rademacher WMH, Hielema A, Wishaw SBP, van Diermen DE, de Lange J, et al. Oral adverse effects: Drug-induced tongue disorders. Oral Diseases. 2021;**27**:1528-1541. DOI: 10.1111/odi.13680

[80] Li Y, Choi H, Leung K, Jiang F, Graham DY, Leung WK. Global prevalence of *Helicobacter pylori* infection between 1980 and 2022: A systematic review and meta-analysis. The Lancet Gastroenterology & Hepatology. 2023;**8**:553-564. DOI: 10.1016/S2468-1253(23)00070-5

[81] Elbehiry A, Marzouk E, Aldubaib M, Abalkhail A, Anagreyyah S, Anajirih N, et al. *Helicobacter pylori* infection: Current status and future

prospects on diagnostic, therapeutic and control challenges. Antibiotics (Basel). 2023;**12**:191. DOI: 10.3390/antibiotics12020191

[82] Rolfo C, Denninghoff V. Globalization of precision medicine programs in lung cancer—A health system challenge. The Lancet Regional Health - Europe. 2023;**36**:100819. DOI: 10.1016/j.lanepe.2023.100819

[83] Usui Y, Taniyama Y, Endo M, Koyanagi YN, Kasugai Y, Oze I, et al. *Helicobacter pylori*, homologous-recombination genes, and gastric cancer. The New England Journal of Medicine. 2023;**388**:1181-1190. DOI: 10.1056/NEJMoa2211807

[84] Paes Dutra JA, Gonçalves Carvalho S, Soares de Oliveira A, Borges Monteiro JR, Rodrigues Pereira de Oliveira Borlot J, Tavares Luiz M, et al. Microparticles and nanoparticles-based approaches to improve oral treatment of *Helicobacter pylori* infection. Critical Reviews in Microbiology. 2023;**28**:1-22. DOI: 10.1080/1040841X.2023.2274835

[85] Noszka M, Strzałka A, Muraszko J, Kolenda R, Meng C, Ludwig C, et al. Profiling of the *Helicobacter pylori* redox switch HP1021 regulon using a multi-omics approach. Nature Communications. 2023;**14**:6715. DOI: 10.1038/s41467-023-42364-6

Chapter 7

Dynamic Changes of Host Immune Response during *Helicobacter pylori*-Induced Gastric Carcinogenesis

Meiling Zhou, Jing Zhang, Weiwei Fu and Shigang Ding

Abstract

Helicobacter pylori infection is identified as a primary risk factor for gastric cancer (GC). Chronic inflammation is usually induced by *H. pylori* infection and accompanied by inherent immune disorders. According to Correa's model, gastritis could progress to premalignant lesions, such as intestinal metaplasia and dysplasia, and ultimately GC. The interaction of *H. pylori* with the gastric mucosa leads to the recruitment of immune cells, including dendritic (DC) cells, natural killer (NK) cells, and T and B lymphocytes, and triggers inflammatory response with cytokine production, which results in the pathogenesis of stomach. The balance between inflammation and immunity is important to gastric cancer development. However, the dynamic change of immune response during the transition from normal to metaplasia to dysplasia and GC is largely undefined. In this review, we summarized the involvement of key immune cells during GC progression, aiming to help identify inflection points and associated biomarkers for early GC detection, diagnosis, and therapies.

Keywords: *Helicobacter pylori*, gastric cancer, immune response, diagnosis, therapy

1. Introduction

The lifetime risk of gastric cancer in patients with *Helicobacter pylori* infection is 1–5%, depending on ethnicity and environmental factors [1]. Some populations have an increased risk of gastric cancer after *H. pylori* infection, which can be attributed to genetics, housing status, and dietary habits, such as increased consumption of salty or pickled foods in East Asian populations. According to the global burden of cancer attributable to infections in 2018 [2], chronic tissue damage with necrosis and regeneration carries an increased cancer risk, especially chronic gastritis caused by *H. pylori* infection. Characteristics of multiple carcinomas suggest that immunologic factors modulate susceptibility to gastric tumors. Nowadays, a significant number of studies have found that *H. pylori* infection is closely related to the occurrence and development of some gastrointestinal diseases, including chronic active gastritis, peptic ulcer, gastric cancer, and gastric mucosa-associated lymphoid lymphoma

(MALT). The pathogenic mechanism of *H. pylori* infection is very complex; in addition to the damage to the gastric mucosa caused by *H. pylori*'s own kinetic apparatus, adhesion properties, and various virulence factors and host genetics, there are also inflammatory and immune responses induced by *H. pylori* infection. During *H. pylori* infection, several cytokines, such as interferon (IFN) and interleukins (IL), play a crucial role in regulating immune and inflammatory responses. In this paper, we reviewed the immunological mechanisms of immune cells and immune molecules in the pathogenesis of gastric mucosa during *H. pylori* infections.

2. *H. pylori* infection associated with T cells

2.1 T helper (Th) cell-mediated gastric mucosal inflammation

$CD4^+$ T cells play a critical role in the immune response elicited during *H. pylori* infection, and Th1 cells undergo the earliest polarized proliferation among them. $CD4^+$ T cells have two primary functions: to promote the inflammatory response and antibody production by B cells. Th1 cells secrete IFN-γ and IL-2 to enhance antigen presentation and to promote bactericidal action by macrophages. Th2 cells secrete IL-4, IL-5, and IL-13. These can promote B-cell proliferation and the production of antibodies. We elaborated on the change of immune cells and how these cells act as a protective factor or cause damage to the gastric mucosa after *H. pylori* infection.

H. pylori can induce Th1 cell response early during acute infection [3]. Additionally, the Th1 cell response was activated by the gastric mucosa dendritic cells in humans [4]. CagY, an *H. pylori* protein, can drive both B-cell proliferation and T-cell activation in gastric MALT lymphomas [5]. They have upregulated the mRNA expression of Notch1 involved in the differentiation of Th1 cells during *H. pylori* infection. *H. pylori* activates the Th1-Th2 response, activating B cells associated with the Th1 response and the Th2-specific antibody IgG1 [6]. Although earlier studies showed a protective factor for Th2 response in protection from *H. pylori* infection, more new reports suggested that protection from *H. pylori* is related to the progression of Th1 responses, which are accompanied by the high expression of IFN-γ and IL-12 and elevated IgG2a/IgG1 ratio as well. Formulations containing rCagA promote a Th1 response and induce Th1/Th2 balance through elevating IL-4, IL-10, and TGF-β levels, which were in line with the proliferation of spleen cells [6].

Th17, a newly identified $CD4^+$ T-cell subtype expressing IL-17A, IL-17F, IL-21, and the chemokine CCL20, as well as the transcription factor RORγt, is involved in the gastric mucosal inflammatory response to *H. pylori* infection. Studies proved that the Th17 response could effectively protect against *H. pylori* infection if mice were immunized with inactive *H. pylori* [7]. In patients with peptic ulcers infected with different bacterial types of *H. pylori*, $CD4^+$ T cells increased. Increased regulatory T-cell activity can reduce the Th17/IL-17 mediated mucosal immune response in the stomach, while Th17 cut can reduce neutrophil accumulation and decrease inflammation in *H. pylori-infected* children [8]. A series of cytokines and transcription factors can regulate the differentiation and function of Th17. More detailed research can be found in this influencing review [9].

Th22 cells and IL-22 play a proinflammatory role in infectious disease [10]. After *H. pylori* infection, IL-22 can inhibit epithelial cell apoptosis and promote epithelial proliferation and regeneration [11], exerting tissue-protective effects regulated by IL-17A [12].

Although *H. pylori* infection of the gastric mucosa can cause Th cells and the inflammatory factors they secrete to accumulate in large numbers and cause disease, the gastric mucosal tissues continue to be damaged after the eradication of *H. pylori*.

2.2 Regulatory T-cell mediated gastric mucosal tolerance

Regulatory T cells (Tregs) are characterized by high levels of CD25, low levels of CD127, and inhibitory cytokines (e.g., IL-10 and the transcription factor Foxp3). They are essential in regulating cellular immune response and maintaining autoimmune tolerance. Tregs inhibit antigen-induced immune reactions, and disordered Treg activation induced by microbial antigens may be a mechanism by which *H. pylori* evades host immune attack. CagA, γ-glutamyl transpeptidase (γGT), vacuolar cytotoxin A (VacA), etc., from *H. pylori,* triggered the differentiation of tolerogenic dendritic cells (DCs), resulting in a bias of Treg cells toward a Th response. γGT, VacA, and arginase inhibited the proliferation of $CD4^+$ and $CD8^+$ T cells [13].

Tregs, $CD4^+CD25^+Foxp3^+$ T cells, are essential in regulating the cellular immune response and maintaining autoimmune tolerance. Tregs negatively regulate the immune response mainly in two ways: one is to inhibit the activation of the target cells directly, and the other is to secrete cytokines, such as TGF-β and IL-10, to inhibit the immune response. In addition, Tregs can hinder the immune response induced by antigens and antibodies, and the abnormal activation of Tregs induced by microbial antigens may be one of the mechanisms by which *H. pylori* evades host immune attack [14]. The expression levels of $CD4^+$ T cells, $Foxp3^+$ Treg cells, and TGF-β1 were higher in children infected with *H. pylori*, and the number of $Foxp3^+$ Treg cells and the expression of TGF-β1 inflammatory factors were positively correlated with having *H. pylori* infection. The results suggest that Treg cells may play an essential role in the persistent infection of gastric mucosa by *H. pylori* [15]. An increased number of Treg cells increases the chances of *H. pylori* infection in children. The two immune cells, Treg and Th, are in equilibrium in the normal state of the organism. In contrast, increased secretion of Treg inhibits the Th-mediated inflammatory response when *H. pylori* infects the organism, which is an essential reason for the involvement of Treg in the pathogenesis of *H. pylori* infection [16]. Among *H. pylori*-infected people, a large amount of Treg accumulates in their gastric mucosa when Treg exerts an immunosuppressive function. Researchers found that two conditions are required for this phenomenon to occur. First, chemokines attract Treg to migrate from the bloodstream to the gastric mucosa; second, Treg can express chemokine receptors and some adhesion molecules. It was further found that chemokine receptor 6 (CCR6) expressed by gastric mucosal epithelial cells can combine with its ligand chemokine CCL20 to elicit immune responses, and the immunoreactivity of *H. pylori* can cause *H. pylori* to express a large amount of CCL20. At the same time, the virulence factor cagPAI can make *H. pylori* express a large amount of CCL20. *H. pylori*'s virulence factor, cagPAI, can cause *H. pylori* to express CCL20 in large quantities [17].

Although *H. pylori* establishes an immune-tolerant environment to some degree, proinflammatory signaling molecules can still initiate systemic and local T-cell inflammatory immune responses to damage gastric mucosal tissues. In the research of gastric cancers associated with *H. pylori*, it would be essential to emphasize the crosstalk of EPHA2 with other RTKs and with different signaling pathways that are well-known driving factors of carcinogenesis and tumor aggressiveness, such as EGFR, MET, and the WNT/β-catenin pathway [18].

2.3 Cytotoxic T-lymphocyte-mediated gastric mucosal inflammation

H. pylori can induce the host $CD4^+$ T-cell immune responses to provide protection, but less is known of $CD8^+$ T-cell responses. $CD8^+$ T cells have long been considered unrelated to the immune response to *H. pylori*. Still, some studies on the characterization of *H. pylori*-associated $CD4^+$ T cells have also referred to the infiltration of gastric mucosa by $CD8^+$ T cells [19]. In *H. pylori* infection, early mucosal T-cell immune response is dominated by $CD8^+$ T cells to control pathogens at the cost of increased tissue inflammation; $CD8^+$ T cells are later overtaken by $CD4^+$ T cells. *H. pylori*-induced gastric $CD8^+$T cells display a tissue-resident memory (T_{RM}) phenotype (T^+_{RM} phenotype) [20]. A research team infected C57BL/6 mice with the pathogenic CagA-proficient *H. pylori* strain PMSS1 at different periods and analyzed single-cell suspensions of the gastric mucosa *via* flow cytometry. Urease subunit B (UreB) is a conserved and critical virulence factor of *H. pylori*. The peripheral blood mononuclear cells (PBMCs) collected from *H. pylori*-infected individuals were stimulated with recombinant UreB (rUreB) *in vitro* to detect specific $CD8^+$ T-cell responses after coculturing with rUreB-pulsed autologous human monocyte-derived dendritic cells (hMDCs) [21]. $CD8^+$ T cells could play an inflammatory scavenging role and kill bacteria in the absence of $CD4^+$ T-cell immunoprotection in mice infected with *H. pylori*, such as in the case of *H. pylori*-infected GK1.5 (anti-CD4)-treated mice. *H. pylori*-infected *MHC-II* knockout mice (both lacked $CD4^+$ T cells) had significant accumulation of $CD8^+$ T cells in the gastric mucosa and had severe gastric mucosal injury, suggesting that $CD8^+$ T cells may mediate the gastric mucosal inflammatory response [22]. Moreover, the researcher established an animal experimental model of *H. pylori*-infected pigs by gavage. The histopathology of the gastric mucosa was similar to that of *H. pylori*-infected humans. The expression of immune molecules such as the marker protein T-bet, CD16, perforin, and granzyme of $CD8^+$ cytotoxic T lymphocytes (CTL) was high, which suggests that CTL mediated gastric mucosal inflammation when the body was subject to *H. pylori* invasion. Thus, $CD8^+$ T cells might mediate gastric mucosal inflammation when *H. pylori* infects the body. CTL-mediated gastric mucosal immune response was predominant when *H. pylori* invaded the organism [23]. *Helicobacter* urease suppresses cytotoxic $CD8^+$ T-cell responses through activating Myh9-dependent induction of PD-L1 [24].

3. *H. pylori* infection associated with B cells

The primary function of B cells is to produce antibodies to mediate the humoral immune response. When *H. pylori* invades the gastric mucosa, B cells limit the invasion and metastasis of *H. pylori* by secreting antibodies to confine *H. pylori* to a specific lesion. The proliferative effect of $CD8^+$ T cells in the blood of patients infected with *H. pylori* by flow cytometry found that B cells could stimulate the increase of $CD8^+$ T cells after the binding of *H. pylori* to the gastric mucosa. The results suggested that this may be one of the mechanisms by which B cells are involved in the fight against *H. pylori* infection and mediate the inflammatory response of gastric mucosal tissues. Regulatory B cells, similar to Treg, can mediate the inflammatory immune response to *H. pylori* infection of the gastric mucosa [25]. A research team produced a C57BL/6 mouse model infected with *H. pylori* Sydney strain (HPSS1) by gavage and found that $Foxp3^+$ Treg and IL-10-secreting regulatory B cells (IL-10, HPSS1, HPSS1, HPSS1, HPSS1, HPSS1, HPSS1, HPSS1, HPSS1, HPSS1, HPSS1, and IL-10-secreting regulatory B cells (IL-10) were the most critical factors in the inflammatory response. The higher number of Foxp3⁺ Treg and IL-10⁺ B cells (the earlier increase of IL-10⁺ B cells compared with Foxp3⁺ Treg) suggested that IL-10⁺ B cells could allow *H. pylori* to escape from the attack at the early stage of infection and persistently colonize the surface of the gastric mucosa, which could then release inflammatory factors to cause gastric mucosal tissue damage. In addition, IL-10⁺ B cells and Foxp3⁺ Treg content in the small intestine and colon mucosa were significantly increased, suggesting that *H. pylori* infection may cause damage to the mucosa of the small intestine and colon [26]. *H. pylori* deregulates T- and B-cell signaling to trigger immune evasion [27].

4. *H. pylori* infection associated with NK cells

NK cells are a class of nonspecific immune lymphocytes different from T and B cells and directly kill target cells. NK cells regulate the host's immune function by releasing inflammatory factors, such as IFN-γ and TNF-α. Some cytokines, such as IL-12 and TNF-α, can regulate NK cell function and induce NK cells to produce IFN-γ. NK cells are the primary effector cells exerting an intrinsic immune response in the gastric mucosa against *H. pylori* infection. Recently, it was found that NK cells could participate in the inflammatory response of *H. pylori*-infected gastric mucosal tissues by releasing IL-12 and IFN-γ, which can be mediated by natural killer group 2, an activating receptor whose ligand (NKG2DL) expression is induced in conditions of cell stress and carcinogenesis transformation [28]. NK cells can secrete IFN-γ, and chronic inflammation in the stomach of *H. pylori*-infected people is mainly characterized by increased IFN-γ secretion, suggesting that NK cells mediate the inflammatory immune response at the same time as clearing *H. pylori* infection. IL-12 can stimulate the production of IFN-γ by NK cells through *H. pylori* or toll-like receptor (TLR)2 ligands [29]. The expression of the costimulatory molecule CD86 and the proliferation of CD56⁺ NK cells were associated with high-grade MALT at the early stage of *H. pylori* infection, suggesting that CD56⁺ NK cells may be involved in the pathogenesis of high-grade gastric MALT lymphoma.

5. *H. pylori* infection associated with dendritic cells

In DCs infected with *H. pylori*, synergistic interactions regulate IL-1β secretion between cagPAI and the TLR2, NOD2, and NLRP3 triad, modulating the inflammatory immune response [30]. DCs are predominantly known for their function as a potent inductive agent of adaptive immunity. DCs exposed to *H. pylori in vitro* or *in vivo* cannot induce T-cell effector functions. Instead, they efficiently induced the expression of the forkhead transcription factor FoxP3, the master regulator of Treg. DC depletion resulted in better infection control and aggravated T-cell-driven immunopathology [31]. Mucosal CD11c dendritic cells are located near the surface of normal gastric epithelium and increase after *H. pylori* infection. The depletion of CD25 Tregs results in an early reduction of *H. pylori* density, correlated with enhanced peripheral *H. pylori*-specific Th17, but not Th1 response [32]. Th17, not Th1, response during *H. pylori* infection is related to a lower level of *H. pylori* colonization in HP-DC-transferred mice. All in all, the mechanism of immune escape of *H. pylori* through the induction of Tregs impedes Th17 immunity [32].

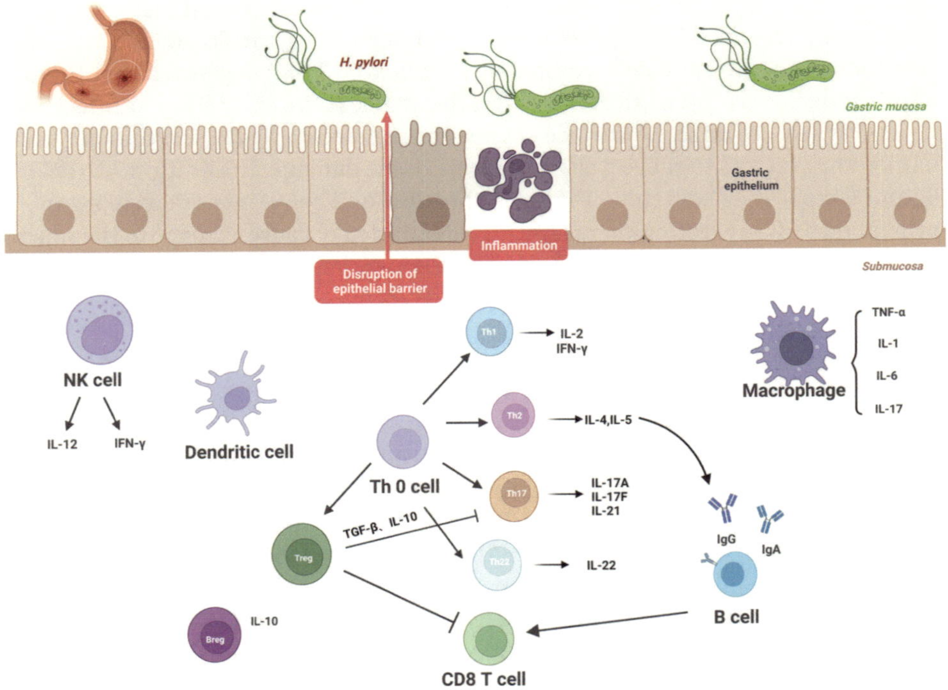

Figure 1.
The change of immune cells in the pathogenesis of gastric mucosa after H. pylori *infections.*

6. *H. pylori* infection associated with macrophages

Macrophages are critical immune cells in the defense of gastric mucosal tissues against *H. pylori* infection, and they mainly work together with reactive oxygen species and reactive nitrogen to clear *H. pylori* through secreted inflammatory cytokines TNF-α, IL-1, IL-6, and IL-17 [33]. When *H. pylori* infects gastric mucosal tissues, macrophages migrate large numbers from the peripheral blood to the infected gastric mucosal tissues for immunomodulation. At the same time, macrophages secrete inflammatory factors that damage the gastric mucosal tissues. BAFF is a pivotal cytokine that impacts the activity of both innate and adaptive immune cells. The expression of IL-17 and BAFF was higher in chronic gastritis patients infected with *H. pylori*, and BAFF cytokines released by macrophages not only altered immune cell activity but also could promote Th17 proliferation, suggesting that macrophages could elicit gastric mucosal inflammatory immune responses through the BAFF/Th17 signaling pathway [34]. The correlation between the immune cells with *H. pylori* infection that are referred to the above is summarized in the **Figure 1**.

7. *H. pylori* infection associated with immune molecules

We will elaborate on the membrane molecular, cytokine, and signal pathway related to *H. pylori* infection which are summarized in the **Table 1**. Toll-like receptor (TLR)-mediated sensing of microbial molecular patterns and corresponding signaling is one of the primary innate immune mechanisms against intruding pathogens. TLRs also play a significant role in innate and adaptive immune responses against

	H. pylori infection	Gastric cancer
Cell types	CD4⁺T cell, CD8⁺T cell, NK cell, B cell, Macrophage, DC	CD4⁺T cell, CD8⁺T cell, B cell, Tumor-Associated Macrophages
Molecules	TLR2, TLR, TLR10, B7H3, SOCS3, CCR2, CXCL2, MMP10, ITGB1	PD-L1, FGFR4, MMPs, CTLA-4, CD44
	IL23, IL33, BAFF, T cell derived cytokines	IL6, IL-10, IL-17A
	STAT3, NF-κB, NLRP3, MyD88	STAT1, STAT3, NF-κB

Table 1.
The dynamic change of immune and non-immune cells during H. pylori *infection and gastric cancer.*

H. pylori. The concentration of TLR2 and TLR4 is higher in *H. pylori*-positive participants compared to the control group [35]. TLR2, TLR4, and TLR10 can shape the cytokine and chemokine release of *H. pylori*-infected human DCs [36]. *H. pylori* infection induces IL-10 secretion in DCs, which activates STAT3, thereby modulating DC maturation and reducing IL-1β secretion [37]. *H. pylori* cytotoxin-associated gene A (Cag A) impairs human dendritic cell maturation and function through IL-10-mediated activation of STAT3 [38]. STAT3 links IL-22 signaling in intestinal epithelial cells to modulate mucosal wound healing [39].

A search team found a new regulatory mechanism employed by *H. pylori* to influence the type of the T-cell response. GEC cocultures and anti-B7-H3 blocking Ab confirmed that the induction of Th2 is mediated by B7-H3 and associated exclusively with an *H. pylori* gastritis strain, not cancer or ulcer strains [40]. High levels of SOCS3 in DCs dampen PD-L1 expression in DCs, which drives T-cell proliferation [41]. CagA interacts with ITGB1, causing gastric mucosa cells to produce IL-8. ITGB1 deficiency can inhibit phosphorylation and activation of p38 and ERK1/2 by CagA [42].

Helicobacter pylori-induced IL-33 modulates mast cell responses and favors bacterial growth [43]. IL-33 can limit immunopathology by promoting T helper 2 immune response. *H. pylori* activates NF-κB signaling *via* the pathogen recognition molecule nucleotide-binding oligomerization domain-containing protein 1 (NOD1) and its receptor to promote and process IL-33 [44]. Mice lacking expression of the CCL2 receptor CCR2 are incapable of responding to *H. pylori* infection [45]. One of the consequences of NF-κB activation in gastric epithelial cells is the production of chemokine CCL2, which serves as a central chemokine attracting myeloid cells to infectious tissues [46]. After *H. pylori* infection, IL-23-induced Th22 cells are rapidly increased in the gastric mucosa, and Th22 can secrete IL-22, which increases CXCL2 production by the gastric mucosa. CXCL2 was combined with its corresponding receptors, leading to migrating myeloid-derived suppressor cells (MDSCs) toward the gastric epithelium. In response to IL-22 induction, MDSCs produce the proinflammatory factors, calgranulin A (S100A8) and S100A9, and directly inhibit the development of Th1 cells, leading to gastritis progression [10]. Moreover, through activation of the signaling pathway of the ERK, *H. pylori* synergistically promotes the production of matrix metalloproteinases (MMPs), especially MMP-10, in gastric epithelial cells. According to former research, MMP-10 can stimulate bacterial colonization by inhibiting the production of antimicrobial peptides in gastric epithelial cells. In addition, MMP-10 also induces gastric epithelial cells to secrete the chemokine CXCL16, which recruits $CD8^+$ T cells to the gastric mucosa and exacerbates the inflammatory response [47]. Also, NLRP3−/−mice cannot activate Treg responses to *H. pylori* and control the infection more effectively than wild-type mice. The results demonstrate NLRP3 is crucial to Treg development and suppression of Th1 responses. Besides, they emphasized the inflammasome-independent function of NLRP3 in DC evolution and immune regulation [45]. *H. pylori* activates different TLR/MyD88 signaling pathways, initiating immune responses that lead to different responses and resultant cascades. This differential pathway activation may depend on the type of *H. pylori* ligand, host TLR source, and species, recruited MyD88 and its downstream molecules, or other host-related factors, even related to different models of TLR ectopic expression [48].

8. Dynamic changes in gastric cancer

Chronic *H. pylori* infection causes long-lasting inflammation in the stomach, which can lead to several possible conditions, including atrophic gastritis (thinning of the stomach lining caused by long-term inflammation) and certain types of stomach (gastric) cancer, particularly gastric adenocarcinoma and gastric mucosa-associated lymphoid tissue (MALT) lymphoma, which is a rare type of non-Hodgkin lymphoma. After elaborating on the relative immune cells and molecules of *H. pylori* infection, we will demonstrate how these immune cells and molecules influence gastric cancer development.

Compared with the normal tissue, Treg cells in gastric cancer increased remarkably [49]. However, relevant transcriptional regulators still need more research to identify [50].

Kynureninase (KYNU), a biomarker of tumor-associated macrophages, is related to the immunosuppressive microenvironment in gastric cancer [51], suggesting the involvement of macrophages in GC. Moreover, converting M2-type TAMs back into M1-type (reprogramming of TAMs) is effective in antitumor therapy in tumor microenvironment (TME) [52]. Cyclase-associated protein 2 (CAP2) promotes gastric cancer metastasis by mediating the interaction between tumor cells and tumor-associated macrophages. M2 macrophage-derived TGFβ1 can influence the activation of M2 macrophage by a TGF β1/JUN/CAP2 positive-feedback loop [53].

H. pylori protein, CagY, can drive both B-cell proliferation and T-cell activation in gastric MALT lymphomas [5]. As to the cytokine levels of gastric cancer, a meta-analysis explored the association between proinflammatory cytokines and GC, of which 61 studies investigating cytokine serum levels were included [54]. They found that patients with GC were found to have significantly elevated levels of IL-6, IL-7, IL-10, IL-12, and TNF-α. IL-6 is one of the most crucial inflammatory cytokines in the action of *H. pylori*-accompanied gastric cancer. From the mechanism perspective, IL-6 activates gastric inflammation and stimulates a proliferative response of the gastric cell. However, long-lasted gastric injury leads to the development of chronic gastritis and inflammation-induced gastric cancer [55]. During atrophic gastritis to dysplasia to gastric cancer, CD44 is significantly increased in individuals, which is related to the IFN-γ production [56]. STAT3 is a proinflammatory oncogenic transcription factor that mediates tumor initiation and progression in several cancer types, including gastric cancer [57]. In *H. pylori*-induced gastritis and gastric carcinogenesis, *H. pylori*-induced STAT3 activation is mediated, at least in part, through ROS-induced upregulation of IL-6 expression [58]. Macrophages after *H. pylori* infection can release cytokine BAFF. BAFF can drive Th17 responses both indirectly by creating a pro-Th17 cytokine milieu through the involvement of innate immune cells and directly *via* the differentiation of T cells toward the specific profile [34]. A recent study shows that IL-17A promotes gastric carcinogenesis, in part, by regulating the IL-17RC/NF-κB/NOX1 pathway [59]. *H. pylori*-induced activation of STAT1 and PD-L1 expression may prevent immune surveillance in the gastric mucosa, allowing premalignant lesions to progress to gastric cancer [60]. Various pathogen-associated molecular patterns (PAMPs) derived from bacteria can bind to different TLRS. After *H. pylori* infection, pathogen-associated molecular patterns (PAMPs) derived from bacteria can attach to different TLRs. When TLR recruits IRAK, TRAF88, and TAK6 to activate the IKK complex and phosphorylate IκB, TLR mediates MYD1-dependent pathways that induce downstream NF-κB programs to promote inflammation and immune responses [48].

Fibroblast growth factor receptors (FGFRs) are a gene family of transmembrane tyrosine kinase receptors that activate critical downstream signaling pathways [61]. FGFR4 overexpression is relevant to the biology of gastric cancer. Also, FGFR4 protects gastric cancer cells from apoptosis during *H. pylori* infection [62]. Moreover, the migration and invasion of GC are mainly associated with MMP2, MMP9 [63], IL-1β [64], and CXCL8 [65]. The **Table 1** summarizes the molecules involved in the *H. pylori* infection and gastric cancer process.

9. Conclusion

Recently, there has been prominent progress in accessing the pathogenesis, diagnosis, and treatment of *H. pylori* infection. This has led to a substantial decline in the incidence of peptic ulcers and a distinct potential for preventing gastric cancer. TME also featured a variety of inflammatory cytokines and chemokines, including CXCL2, IL-1, IL-6, GM-CSF, and IFN-γ. Intricate interactions between immune cells with cytokines and cancer cells promote cancer progression [48]. In the gastric mucosa, *H. pylori* promotes the differentiation of tolerogenic DCs, M2 macrophages, and Treg cells; inhibits the Th1/Th17 response; and/or sequesters $CD8^+$ T cells [13]. *H. pylori* and cytokine gene variants as predictors of premalignant gastric lesions have been emphasized. An association between anti-*H. pylori* IgG titers and the TLR1/6/10 locus with top SNP rs12233670 was demonstrated in the discovery phase using the fixed-effect model [66]. Throughout some meta-analyses, IL-6 is one of the most critical inflammatory cytokines in the action of *H. pylori*-associated gastric cancer. Maybe it is too early to either confirm or rule out a role for TLR1 loci as genetic risk factors for *H. pylori* infection. Inherited variation of the TLR1/6/10 locus confers immunologic cellular consequences, but high heterogeneity, cohort differences, and antibody decay likely prevent the replication of previous associations with anti-*H. pylori* IgG. In gastric cancer, *H. pylori* infection increases the expression of tyrosine kinases, such as FYN, AKT3, MAPK, YES, SRC, PDK1, and mTOR. *H. pylori* activates and secretes proinflammatory cytokines *via* activated signaling pathways, causing gastric cancer development. The inflammatory immune response induced by *H. pylori* cannot completely clear *H. pylori* and, worse still, induce localized inflammatory damage to the gastric mucosa. Relevant dynamic changes of host immune response during the *H. pylori*-induced gastric carcinogenesis deserve more investigation.

Acknowledgements

This work was supported by the National Natural Science Foundation of China (Grant Number 82270592).

Authorship

W.F. conceived the proposal. M.Z. prepared the manuscript. W.F., J.Z., and S.D. revised the manuscript.

Disclosures

The authors declare no conflicts of interest.

Abbreviations

BAFF, B-cell	activating factor
CagA	cytotoxin-associated gene A
cagPAI	cag pathogenicity island
CAP2	cyclase-associated protein 2
CCR6	chemokine receptor 6
CTL	cytotoxic T lymphocyte
DC	dendritic cell
ERK	extracellular signal-regulated kinases
FGFRs	fibroblast growth factor receptors
GC	gastric cancer
γGT	γ-glutamyl transpeptidase
hMDCs	human monocyte-derived dendritic cells
HPSS1	*H. pylori* sydney strain 1
H. pylori	*Helicobacter pylori*
IFN	interferon
IL	interleukins
IRAK	interleukin-1 receptor (IL-1R)-associated kinase
KYNU	kynureninase
MALT	mucosa-associated lymphoid tissue
MDSCs	myeloid-derived suppressor cells
MMPs	matrix metalloproteinases
MyD88	myeloid differentiation primary response 88
NLRP3	NLR family pyrin domain containing 3
NOD1	nucleotide-binding oligomerization domain-containing protein 1
NK	natural killer
PAMPs	pathogen-associated molecular patterns
PBMCs	peripheral blood mononuclear cells
TAMs	tumor-associated macrophages
TGF-β	transforming growth factor β
Th	T helper
TLR	toll-like receptor
TME	tumor microenvironment
Tregs	regulatory T cells
T + $_{RM}$ phenotype	tissue-resident memory (T_{RM}) phenotype;
UreB	urease subunit B
VacA	vacuolar cytotoxin A.

Author details

Meiling Zhou[1,2], Jing Zhang[1,2], Weiwei Fu[1,2*] and Shigang Ding[1,2*]

1 Department of Gastroenterology, Peking University Third Hospital, Beijing, China

2 Beijing Key Laboratory for Helicobacter pylori Infection and Upper Gastrointestinal Diseases, Beijing, China

*Address all correspondence to: fuweiwei1999@163.com
and dingshigang222@163.com

References

[1] Liou J-M, Malfertheiner P, Lee Y-C, Sheu B-S, Sugano K, Cheng H-C, et al. Screening and eradication of *Helicobacter pylori* for gastric cancer prevention: The Taipei global consensus. Gut. 2020;**69**:2093-2112. DOI: 10.1136/gutjnl-2020-322368

[2] de Martel C, Georges D, Bray F, Ferlay J, Clifford GM. Global burden of cancer attributable to infections in 2018: A worldwide incidence analysis. The Lancet Global Health. 2020;**8**:e180-e190. DOI: 10.1016/S2214-109X(19)30488-7

[3] Mattapallil JJ, Dandekar S, Canfield DR, Solnick JV. A predominant Th1 type of immune response is induced early during acute *Helicobacter pylori* infection in rhesus macaques. Gastroenterology. 2000;**118**:307-315. DOI: 10.1016/S0016-5085(00)70213-7

[4] Bimczok D, Clements RH, Waites KB, Novak L, Eckhoff DE, Mannon PJ, et al. Human primary gastric dendritic cells induce a Th1 response to *H. pylori*. Mucosal Immunology. 2010;**3**:260-269. DOI: 10.1038/mi.2010.10

[5] Della, Bella C, Soluri MF, Puccio S, Benagiano M, Grassi A, Bitetti J, et al. The *Helicobacter pylori* CagY protein drives gastric Th1 and Th17 inflammation and B cell proliferation in gastric MALT lymphoma. IJMS. 2021;**22**:9459. DOI: 10.3390/ijms22179459

[6] Paydarnia N, Mansoori B, Esmaeili D, Kazemi T, Aghapour M, Hajiasgharzadeh K, et al. *Helicobacter pylori* recombinant CagA regulates Th1/Th2 balance in a BALB/c murine model. Advanced Pharmaceutical Bulletin. 2020;**10**:264-270. DOI: 10.34172/apb.2020.031

[7] DeLyria ES, Redline RW, Blanchard TG. Vaccination of mice against *H. Pylori* induces a strong Th-17 response and immunity that is neutrophil dependent. Gastroenterology. 2009;**136**:247-256. DOI: 10.1053/j.gastro.2008.09.017

[8] Serrano C, Wright SW, Bimczok D, Shaffer CL, Cover TL, Venegas A, et al. Downregulated Th17 responses are associated with reduced gastritis in *Helicobacter pylori*–infected children. Mucosal Immunology. 2013;**6**:950-959. DOI: 10.1038/mi.2012.133

[9] Dong C. Cytokine regulation and function in T cells. Annual Review of Immunology. 2021;**39**:51-76. DOI: 10.1146/annurev-immunol-061020-053702

[10] Zhuang Y, Cheng P, Liu X, Peng L, Li B, Wang T, et al. A pro-inflammatory role for Th22 cells in *Helicobacter pylori*-associated gastritis. Gut. 2015;**64**:1368-1378. DOI: 10.1136/gutjnl-2014-307020

[11] Aujla SJ, Chan YR, Zheng M, Fei M, Askew DJ, Pociask DA, et al. IL-22 mediates mucosal host defense against gram-negative bacterial pneumonia. Nature Medicine. 2008;**14**:275-281. DOI: 10.1038/nm1710

[12] Sonnenberg GF, Nair MG, Kirn TJ, Zaph C, Fouser LA, Artis D. Pathological versus protective functions of IL-22 in airway inflammation are regulated by IL-17A. Journal of Experimental Medicine. 2010;**207**:1293-1305. DOI: 10.1084/jem.20092054

[13] Oster P, Vaillant L, McMillan B, Velin D. The efficacy of cancer immunotherapies is compromised by *Helicobacter pylori* infection. Frontiers in Immunology. 2022;**13**:899161. DOI: 10.3389/fimmu.2022.899161

[14] Michetti P, Svennerholm A. *Helicobacter pylori* – inflammation, immunity and vaccines. Helicobacter. 2003;**8**:31-35. DOI: 10.1046/j.1523-5378.2003.00164.x

[15] Cho KY, Cho MS, Seo JW. FOXP3+ regulatory T cells in children with *Helicobacter pylori* infection. Pediatric and Developmental Pathology. 2012;**15**:118-126. DOI: 10.2350/11-06-1046-OA.1

[16] Bagheri N, Azadegan-Dehkordi F, Rahimian G, Rafieian-Kopaei M, Shirzad H. Role of regulatory T-cells in different clinical expressions of *Helicobacter pylori* infection. Archives of Medical Research. 2016;**47**:245-254. DOI: 10.1016/j.arcmed.2016.07.013

[17] Leake I. *Helicobacter pylori* induces changes in regulatory T cells. Nature Reviews. Gastroenterology & Hepatology. 2014;**11**:141-141. DOI: 10.1038/nrgastro.2014.13

[18] Arienti C, Pignatta S, Tesei A. Epidermal growth factor receptor family and its role in gastric cancer. Frontiers in Oncology. 2019;**9**:1308. DOI: 10.3389/fonc.2019.01308

[19] Bamford KB, Fan X, Crowe SE, Leary JF, Gourley WK, Luthra GK, et al. Lymphocytes in the human gastric mucosa during *Helicobacter pylori* have a T helper cell 1 phenotype. Gastroenterology. 1998;**114**:482-492. DOI: 10.1016/S0016-5085(98)70531-1

[20] Koch MRA, Gong R, Friedrich V, Engelsberger V, Kretschmer L, Wanisch A, et al. CagA-specific gastric CD8+ tissue-resident T cells control *Helicobacter pylori* during the early infection phase. Gastroenterology. 2023;**164**:550-566. DOI: 10.1053/j.gastro.2022.12.016

[21] Zhang Z, Chen X, Li B, Xia T, Wu X, Wu C. *Helicobacter pylori* induces urease subunit B-specific CD8^{+} T cell responses in infected individuals via cytosolic pathway of cross-presentation. Helicobacter. 2023;**28**:e13005. DOI: 10.1111/hel.13005

[22] Kronsteiner B, Bassaganya-Riera J, Philipson N, Hontecillas R. Novel insights on the role of CD8+ T cells and cytotoxic responses during *Helicobacter pylori* infection. Gut Microbes. 2014;**5**:357-362. DOI: 10.4161/gmic.28899

[23] Kronsteiner B, Bassaganya-Riera J, Philipson C, Viladomiu M, Carbo A, Pedragosa M, et al. *Helicobacter pylori* infection in a pig model is dominated by Th1 and cytotoxic CD8^{+} T cell responses. Infection and Immunity. 2013;**81**:3803-3813. DOI: 10.1128/IAI.00660-13

[24] Wu J, Zhu X, Guo X, Yang Z, Cai Q, Gu D, et al. Helicobacter urease suppresses cytotoxic CD8^{+} T-cell responses through activating Myh9-dependent induction of PD-L1. International Immunology. 2021;**33**:491-504. DOI: 10.1093/intimm/dxab044

[25] Azem J, Svennerholm A-M, Lundin BS. B cells pulsed with *Helicobacter pylori* antigen efficiently activate memory CD8^{+} T cells from *H. Pylori*-infected individuals. Clinical Immunology. 2006;**118**:284-291. DOI: 10.1016/j.clim.2005.09.011

[26] Wei L, Wang J, Liu Y. Prior to Foxp3^{+} regulatory T-cell induction, interleukin-10-producing B cells expand after *Helicobacter pylori* infection. Pathogens Disease. 2014;**72**:45-54. DOI: 10.1111/2049-632X.12182

[27] Reyes VE, Peniche AG. *Helicobacter Pylori* Deregulates T and B Cell Signaling to Trigger Immune Evasion. In Molecular Mechanisms of Inflammation: Induction, Resolution and Escape by *Helicobacter pylori*. In: Backert S, editor. Current

Topics in Microbiology and Immunology. Vol. 421. Cham: Springer International Publishing; 2019. pp. 229-265, ISBN 978-3-030-15137-9

[28] Hernández C, Toledo-Stuardo K, García-González P, Garrido-Tapia M, Kramm K, Rodríguez-Siza JA, et al. Heat-killed *helicobacter pylori* upregulates NKG2D ligands expression on gastric adenocarcinoma cells via toll-like receptor 4. Helicobacter. 2021;**26**:e12812. DOI: 10.1111/hel.12812

[29] Kuo S-H. Expression of CD86 and increased infiltration of NK cells are associated with *Helicobacter pylori*-dependent state of early stage high-grade gastric MALT lymphoma. WJG. 2005;**11**:4357. DOI: 10.3748/wjg.v11.i28.4357

[30] Kim D, Park J, Franchi L, Backert S, Núñez G. The cag pathogenicity island and interaction between TLR 2/NOD 2 and NLRP 3 regulate IL-1β production in *Helicobacter pylori* infected dendritic cells. European Journal of Immunology. 2013;**43**:2650-2658. DOI: 10.1002/eji.201243281

[31] Oertli M, Sundquist M, Hitzler I, Engler DB, Arnold IC, Reuter S, et al. DC-derived IL-18 drives Treg differentiation, murine *helicobacter pylori*–specific immune tolerance, and asthma protection. The Journal of Clinical Investigation. 2012;**122**:1082-1096. DOI: 10.1172/JCI61029

[32] Kao JY, Zhang M, Miller MJ, Mills JC, Wang B, Liu M, et al. *Helicobacter pylori* immune escape is mediated by dendritic cell–induced Treg skewing and Th17 suppression in mice. Gastroenterology. 2010;**138**:1046-1054. DOI: 10.1053/j.gastro.2009.11.043

[33] Slomiany BL, Slomiany A. Modulation of gastric mucosal inflammatory responses to *helicobacter pylori* via ghrelin-induced protein kinase Cδ tyrosine phosphorylation. Inflammopharmacology. 2014;**22**:251-262. DOI: 10.1007/s10787-014-0206-z

[34] Munari F, Fassan M, Capitani N, Codolo G, Vila-Caballer M, Pizzi M, et al. Cytokine BAFF released by *helicobacter pylori* – Infected macrophages triggers the Th17 response in human chronic gastritis. The Journal of Immunology. 2014;**193**:5584-5594. DOI: 10.4049/jimmunol.1302865

[35] Kareem RA, Kadhim Baqer L. Immunological role of toll like receptor markers (TLR2 and TLR4) In patients with *helicobacter pylori* infection At Basrah, Iraq. Archives of Razi Institute. 2022;**78**(2):601-609. DOI: 10.22092/ari.2022.359715.2458

[36] Neuper T, Frauenlob T, Sarajlic M, Posselt G, Wessler S, Horejs-Hoeck J. TLR2, TLR4 and TLR10 shape the cytokine and chemokine release of *H. pylori*-infected human DCs. IJMS. 2020;**21**:3897. DOI: 10.3390/ijms21113897

[37] Rizzuti D, Ang M, Sokollik C, Wu T, Abdullah M, Greenfield L, et al. *Helicobacter pylori* inhibits dendritic cell maturation via Interleukin-10-mediated activation of the signal transducer and activator of transcription 3 pathway. Journal of Innate Immunity. 2015;7:199-211. DOI: 10.1159/000368232

[38] Kaebisch R, Mejías-Luque R, Prinz C, Gerhard M. *Helicobacter pylori* cytotoxin-associated Gene a impairs human dendritic cell maturation and function through IL-10–mediated activation of STAT3. The Journal of Immunology. 2014;**192**:316-323. DOI: 10.4049/jimmunol.1302476

[39] Pickert G, Neufert C, Leppkes M, Zheng Y, Wittkopf N, Warntjen M, et al.

STAT3 links IL-22 signaling in intestinal epithelial cells to mucosal wound healing. Journal of Experimental Medicine. 2009;**206**:1465-1472. DOI: 10.1084/jem.20082683

[40] Lina TT, Gonzalez J, Pinchuk IV, Beswick EJ, Reyes VE. *Helicobacter pylori* elicits B7-H3 expression on gastric epithelial cells: Implications in local T cell regulation and subset development during infection. COR. 2019;**2**:1-12. DOI: 10.31487/j.COR.2019.05.05

[41] Sarajlic M, Neuper T, Vetter J, Schaller S, Klicznik MM, Gratz IK, et al. *H. pylori* modulates DC functions via T4SS/TNFα/P38-dependent SOCS3 expression. Cell Communication and Signaling: CCS. 2020;**18**:160. DOI: 10.1186/s12964-020-00655-1

[42] Mostaghimi T, Bahadoran E, Bakht M, Taheri S, Sadeghi H, Babaei A. Role of lncRNAs in *helicobacter pylori* and Epstein-Barr virus associated gastric cancers. Life Sciences. 2024;**336**:122316. DOI: 10.1016/j.lfs.2023.122316

[43] Lv Y, Teng Y, Mao F, Peng L, Zhang J, Cheng P, et al. *Helicobacter pylori*-induced IL-33 modulates mast cell responses, benefits bacterial growth, and contributes to gastritis. Cell Death & Disease. 2018;**9**:457. DOI: 10.1038/s41419-018-0493-1

[44] Tran LS, Tran D, De Paoli A, D'Costa K, Creed SJ, Ng GZ, et al. NOD1 is required for *helicobacter pylori* induction of IL-33 responses in gastric epithelial cells. Cellular Microbiology. 2018;**20**:e12826. DOI: 10.1111/cmi.12826

[45] Arnold IC, Zhang X, Urban S, Artola-Borán M, Manz MG, Ottemann KM, et al. NLRP3 controls the development of gastrointestinal CD11b + dendritic cells in the steady state and during chronic bacterial infection. Cell Reports. 2017;**21**:3860-3872. DOI: 10.1016/j.celrep.2017.12.015

[46] Zhang X, Arnold IC, Müller A. Mechanisms of persistence, innate immune activation and immunomodulation by the gastric pathogen *helicobacter pylori*. Current Opinion in Microbiology. 2020;**54**:1-10. DOI: 10.1016/j.mib.2020.01.003

[47] Lv Y, Cheng P, Zhang J, Mao F, Teng Y, Liu Y, et al. *Helicobacter pylori* – induced matrix metallopeptidase-10 promotes gastric bacterial colonization and gastritis. Science Advances. 2019;**5**:eaau6547. DOI: 10.1126/sciadv.aau6547

[48] Liu M, Hu Z, Wang C, Zhang Y. The TLR/MyD88 signalling cascade in inflammation and gastric cancer: The immune regulatory network of *helicobacter pylori*. Journal of Molecular Medicine. 2023;**101**:767-781. DOI: 10.1007/s00109-023-02332-5

[49] Sathe A, Grimes SM, Lau BT, Chen J, Suarez C, Huang RJ, et al. Single-cell genomic characterization reveals the cellular reprogramming of the gastric tumor microenvironment. Clinical Cancer Research. 2020;**26**:2640-2653. DOI: 10.1158/1078-0432.CCR-19-3231

[50] Tang F, Du X, Liu M, Zheng P, Liu Y. Anti-CTLA-4 antibodies in cancer immunotherapy: Selective depletion of Intratumoral regulatory T cells or checkpoint blockade? Cell & Bioscience. 2018;**8**:30. DOI: 10.1186/s13578-018-0229-z

[51] Shen K, Chen B, Yang L, Gao W. KYNU as a biomarker of tumor-associated macrophages and correlates with immunosuppressive microenvironment and poor prognosis in gastric cancer. International Journal of Genomics. 2023;**2023**:4662480. DOI: 10.1155/2023/4662480

[52] Shime H, Matsumoto M, Oshiumi H, Tanaka S, Nakane A, Iwakura Y, et al. Toll-like receptor 3 signaling converts tumor-supporting myeloid cells to tumoricidal effectors. Proceedings of the National Academy of Sciences of the United States of America. 2012;**109**:2066-2071. DOI: 10.1073/pnas.1113099109

[53] Zhang G, Gao Z, Guo X, Ma R, Wang X, Zhou P, et al. CAP2 promotes gastric cancer metastasis by mediating the interaction between tumor cells and tumor-associated macrophages. The Journal of Clinical Investigation. 2023;**133**:e166224. DOI: 10.1172/JCI166224

[54] Yu B, Xiang L, Peppelenbosch MP, Fuhler GM. Overlapping cytokines in *H. Pylori* infection and gastric cancer: A tandem meta-analysis. Frontiers in Immunology. 2023;**14**:1125658. DOI: 10.3389/fimmu.2023.1125658

[55] Kuhn KA, Manieri NA, Liu T-C, Stappenbeck TS. IL-6 stimulates intestinal epithelial proliferation and repair after injury. PLoS One. 2014;**9**:e114195. DOI: 10.1371/journal.pone.0114195

[56] Garay J, Piazuelo MB, Majumdar S, Li L, Trillo-Tinoco J, Del Valle L, et al. The homing receptor CD44 is involved in the progression of precancerous gastric lesions in patients infected with *helicobacter pylori* and in development of mucous metaplasia in mice. Cancer Letters. 2016;**371**:90-98. DOI: 10.1016/j.canlet.2015.10.037

[57] Yu H, Lee H, Herrmann A, Buettner R, Jove R. Revisiting STAT3 Signalling in cancer: New and unexpected biological functions. Nature Reviews. Cancer. 2014;**14**:736-746. DOI: 10.1038/nrc3818

[58] Piao J, Lee HG, Kim S, Kim D, Han H, Ngo H, et al. *Helicobacter pylori* activates IL-6-STAT3 signaling in human gastric cancer cells: Potential roles for reactive oxygen species. Helicobacter. 2016;**21**:405-416. DOI: 10.1111/hel.12298

[59] Kang JH, Park S, Rho J, Hong E-J, Cho Y-E, Won Y-S, et al. IL-17A promotes *helicobacter pylori*-induced gastric carcinogenesis via interactions with IL-17RC. Gastric Cancer. 2023;**26**:82-94. DOI: 10.1007/s10120-022-01342-5

[60] Li X, Pan K, Vieth M, Gerhard M, Li W, Mejías-Luque R. JAK-STAT1 signaling pathway is an early response to *helicobacter pylori* infection and contributes to immune escape and gastric carcinogenesis. IJMS. 2022;**23**:4147. DOI: 10.3390/ijms23084147

[61] Katoh M. Fibroblast growth factor receptors as treatment targets in clinical oncology. Nature Reviews. Clinical Oncology. 2019;**16**:105-122. DOI: 10.1038/s41571-018-0115-y

[62] Zhang X, Soutto M, Chen Z, Bhat N, Zhu S, Eissmann MF, et al. Induction of fibroblast growth factor receptor 4 by *helicobacter pylori* via signal transducer and activator of transcription 3 with a feedforward activation loop involving SRC signaling in gastric cancer. Gastroenterology. 2022;**163**:620-636.e9. DOI: 10.1053/j.gastro.2022.05.016

[63] Xu J, Yu Y, He X, Niu N, Li X, Zhang R, et al. Tumor-associated macrophages induce invasion and poor prognosis in human gastric cancer in a cyclooxygenase-2/MMP9-dependent manner. American Journal of Translational Research. 2019;**11**:6040-6054

[64] Zhang J, Fu L, Yasuda-Yoshihara N, Yonemura A, Wei F, Bu L, et al. IL-1β derived from mixed-polarized macrophages activates fibroblasts and synergistically forms a cancer-promoting

microenvironment. Gastric Cancer. 2023;**26**:187-202. DOI: 10.1007/s10120-022-01352-3

[65] Piao H, Fu L, Wang Y, Liu Y, Wang Y, Meng X, et al. A positive feedback loop between gastric cancer cells and tumor-associated macrophage induces malignancy progression. Journal of Experimental & Clinical Cancer Research. 2022;**41**:174. DOI: 10.1186/s13046-022-02366-6

[66] Lam SY, Mommersteeg MC, Yu B, Broer L, Spaander MCW, Frost F, et al. Toll-like receptor 1 locus Re-examined in a genome-wide association study update on anti–*helicobacter pylori* IgG titers. Gastroenterology. 2022;**162**:1705-1715. DOI: 10.1053/j.gastro.2022.01.011

Chapter 8

Complementary Replacement Therapy for Chronic Gastritis

Liu Mi, Liu Weiai, She Chang, Zhou Jingying, Xu Xuan and He Haolong

Abstract

Gastritis, an inflammation of the stomach lining, arises from diverse causes and ranks among the most frequent digestive ailments. It typically falls into two categories based on the speed of onset: acute and chronic gastritis. Patients with acute gastritis are generally managed symptomatically. Meanwhile, those with chronic gastritis experience ongoing discomfort like epigastric pain, belching, and acid reflux, negatively impacting their quality of life. They can benefit from presently approved medical treatments. To alleviate the physical and mental burden of chronic gastritis and enhance life quality, many patients explore complementary and alternative therapies (CAM). A wide array of CAM options exists, but their safety and effectiveness remain uncertain. If supported by robust evidence, these therapies could potentially become part of standard medical practice for treating chronic gastritis. Approaches like Traditional Chinese Medicine, Acupuncture, Tuina, Diet, Exercise, and Psychological Interventions have demonstrated the capacity to ameliorate symptoms and enhance the well-being of chronic gastritis patients. Identifying high-quality evidence regarding efficacy and safety through Randomized Controlled Trials (RCTs) can facilitate the broader integration of CAM in chronic gastritis treatment. This section offers an overview of the most recent clinical trial findings concerning complementary and alternative therapies.

Keywords: gastritis, complementary replacement therapy, chronic gastritis, clinical trials, traditional Chinese medicine

1. Introduction

Chronic gastritis is a prevalent digestive disorder worldwide, categorized mainly as chronic non-atrophic gastritis and chronic atrophic gastritis. Its occurrence is closely linked to factors such as *Helicobacter pylori* infection, unhealthy dietary habits, irregular sleep patterns, and emotional instability. According to the World Health Organization, China has witnessed a staggering 30% incidence rate of chronic gastritis. With improving living standards and an aging population, this condition's prevalence is projected to rise annually. Recurrent chronic gastritis significantly diminishes patients' quality of life and adds to their emotional burden. Furthermore, if left untreated over extended periods, chronic gastritis can progress to gastric cancer, heightening the risk of cancer among affected individuals. Therefore, the effective prevention and treatment of chronic gastritis present a significant and challenging issue in clinical medicine.

While drugs like gastric acid inhibitors, *Helicobacter pylori* eradicators, and gastric mucosal protectors have made substantial contributions to managing common chronic gastritis symptoms, they cannot completely eradicate the condition. Moreover, they may lead to adverse reactions and side effects, including reduced drug tolerance, increased drug dependence, and drug interactions. Consequently, many chronic gastritis patients turn to complementary and alternative therapies alongside conventional medical treatments to alleviate discomfort and enhance their quality of life. Complementary and alternative medicine encompasses a range of diagnostic, therapeutic, and preventive methods outside mainstream medicine. It complements mainstream medical practices and offers approaches that mainstream medicine cannot provide. These categories include alternative medicine systems, spiritual intention therapy, biological-based therapies, body adjustment therapy, and energy therapy. Currently, complementary alternative medicine is widely utilized in the clinical management of chronic gastritis, gaining the trust and favor of both patients and healthcare professionals. Traditional Chinese medicine, with its centuries of development, has amassed a wealth of knowledge and techniques for treating digestive system disorders. It stands as a crucial representative of complementary alternative medicine, incorporating Chinese herbal remedies, acupuncture, tuina massage, dietary therapy, qigong exercises, emotional regulation, and other evidence-based treatments tailored to individual patient conditions. These approaches offer several advantages, such as fewer side effects. Over the past decades, extensive research has explored the potential benefits of complementary alternative therapies in preventing and treating chronic gastritis, laying a scientific foundation for their broader adoption. Many complementary alternative therapies, including qigong, moxibustion, and dietary adjustments, are straightforward and easily integrated into people's daily lives. A comprehensive understanding of these methods enhances patient self-care awareness and provides a valuable reference for patients seeking appropriate treatment options.

This chapter presents the most recent clinical evidence and offers a systematic overview of the current utilization of various complementary alternative therapies for treating chronic gastritis. These therapies encompass Chinese herbal medicine, acupuncture, massage, dietary interventions, exercise, and psychological approaches. The information presented here is not only enlightening but also holds substantial importance for the recovery and enhancement of the quality of life in individuals with chronic gastritis. Additionally, it carries significant implications for advancing research and development in the integration of traditional Chinese medicine with Western medicine. This book caters to a diverse audience, including chronic gastritis patients and their families, healthcare practitioners, and professionals in related fields.

2. Chinese herbal medicine for chronic gastritis

In accordance with traditional Chinese medicine (TCM) principles, chronic gastritis is attributed to imbalances in the Qi mechanism, along with a loss of stomach function and descending. An increasing number of clinical trials have provided compelling evidence for the efficacy of traditional Chinese medicine in the treatment of chronic gastritis. Specifically, it has demonstrated effectiveness in alleviating discomforting symptoms associated with chronic gastritis, such as abdominal distension, abdominal pain, acid reflux, and fatigue. Consequently, it can be considered a dependable complementary therapeutic option that widens the spectrum of treatments available for chronic gastritis.

Tian Guihua, Wu Chuanhong [1], and their team conducted a study involving 20 patients diagnosed with chronic atrophic gastritis of spleen-qi deficiency type. These patients received Sijunzi Decoction continuously for four weeks, leading to noteworthy improvements in clinical discomfort symptoms like abdominal distension and fatigue. Electronic gastroscopy results illustrated that Sijunzi Decoction effectively mitigated gastric mucosa erosion and atrophy in patients with chronic gastritis of spleen-qi deficiency type. The outcomes of the Sijunzi Decoction TCM target network analysis indicate that Radix Astragali can alleviate appetite loss due to spleen deficiency and nourish the spleen and Qi. Rhizoma Atractylodis Macrocephalae, when stir-fried with bran, helps alleviate abdominal distension and increases food intake. Moreover, Poria and honey-fried Radix Glycyrrhizae can alleviate abdominal distension and dull abdominal pain. This study underscores the efficacy of the mentioned traditional Chinese medicine in ameliorating clinical discomfort symptoms associated with chronic gastritis through Qi tonification.

In a study led by Zhao Yushu [2], the clinical effectiveness of Banxia Xiexin Decoction in treating chronic atrophic gastritis with mixed cold and heat syndrome was analyzed. A total of 84 patients with this condition were chosen for the study. After one month of continuous treatment, gastroscopy revealed substantial normalization of the gastric mucosa in patients. The pale areas of the gastric mucosa significantly decreased compared to the pre-treatment condition. The observation group achieved an impressive total effective rate of 95.24%, significantly surpassing the control group. The researcher suggests that including Pinellia in Banxia Xiexin Decoction aids in dampness reduction and minimizes adverse effects, while dried ginger warms the stomach and dispels pathogenic cold. Additionally, Scutellaria baicalensis and Coptis chinensis contribute to heat and dampness elimination, detoxification, and *Codonopsis pilosula* strengthens the spleen and replenishes Qi. The combined effects substantially enhance the clinical effectiveness of patients with chronic gastritis, rendering it a recommended treatment.

Muo-luo-dan, a traditional Chinese medicine preparation comprising Lily, *Ophiopogon japonicus*, Panax notoginseng, Poria cocos, and Atractylodes macrocephala, was investigated for its clinical efficacy in treating chronic atrophic gastritis in a study conducted by Ma Chunlei et al. [3]. This randomized controlled trial involved 128 patients diagnosed with gastric chronic atrophic gastritis confirmed through gastroscopic biopsy. After a 3-month treatment period, patients receiving Muo-luo-dan treatment exhibited significant increases in Gastrin-17 (G-17) and Pepsinogen I (PG I) levels. Furthermore, the degree of atrophy in the gastric intrinsic gland was notably improved in the Muo-luo-dan treatment group compared to the control group. G-17 is a vital gastrointestinal hormone that regulates digestive tract function, while PG I is closely linked to gastric acid secretion and digestive function, effectively reflecting the extent of gastric mucosal damage. This clinical trial provides robust evidence that traditional Chinese medicine Muo-luo-dan effectively reduces gastric mucosal injury and enhances gastric function in chronic atrophic gastritis patients. These improvements are instrumental in alleviating clinical discomfort symptoms and slowing the disease's progression.

Numerous clinical trials have also explored the development of new traditional Chinese medicine preparations for chronic gastritis treatment. Yu Bin et al. [4] conducted an open multicenter clinical trial utilizing Liqi Warming Stomach Granules, developed by Jiangxi Huiren Pharmaceutical, for treating chronic superficial gastritis, involving no fewer than 2000 cases. Liqi Nuanwei Granules, composed of Chinese herbal medicines like Bupleurum Radix, Radix Paeoniae Alba, Galangal, and Rhizoma Cyperi, aimed to observe the improvement in primary symptoms in chronic gastritis patients before and after treatment. After a 4-week treatment period, the results indicated an 89.51% total effective rate in alleviating epigastric pain and other symptoms. Additionally, sub-symptoms such as belching, acid reflux, and appetite loss exhibited significant increases in TCM curative effect scores. This trial provides substantial evidence supporting the definite therapeutic efficacy of traditional Chinese medicine in ameliorating the clinical symptoms of chronic gastritis.

Pingwei Decoction is a commonly used prescription for addressing spleen-stomach disharmony and stomach-related ailments. In a study led by Hu Chunping, Cai Yisheng, and their team, 60 patients with chronic gastritis atrophy and intestinal metaplasia were enrolled to assess the clinical efficacy of Pingwei Decoction [5]. The prescription comprises traditional Chinese medicines such as Malt, Poria cocos, Polygonatum sibiricum, Atractylodes rhizome, *Pinellia ternata*, among others, and was administered once in the morning and once in the evening. Following three months of continuous treatment, the evaluation of treatment outcomes indicated that the treatment group exhibited a significantly higher effective rate of 96.67% compared to the observation group. Gastroscopy findings revealed improvements in the gastric antrum glands and intestinal metaplasia following Pingwei Decoction treatment. Additionally, TCM symptom scores showcased a reduction in epigastric pain, belching, and acid reflux after the intervention. Moreover, serum gastrin test results demonstrated a significant increase in serum gastrin levels post-treatment. These findings robustly support the effectiveness of Pingwei Decoction in managing chronic gastritis, validating its clinical utility. The researcher suggests that Malt in Pingwei Decoction promotes Qi and aids digestion, while Poria cocos and Polygonatum sibiricum fortify the spleen and replenish Qi. Atractylodes rhizome can eliminate dampness and strengthen the spleen, while *Pinellia ternata* reduces adverse effects and alleviates vomiting. The combined action of these components yields a favorable therapeutic effect for chronic gastritis.

In addition to Pingwei Decoction, Modified Sanren Decoction is another empirical prescription for treating spleen and stomach ailments. Guo Xinyi, et al. conducted a study involving 35 patients with chronic non-atrophic gastritis to assess the clinical effectiveness of Modified Sanren Decoction [6]. The primary constituents of this medicine include Almonds, Coix seed, Cardamom seed, Magnolia officinalis, *Pinellia ternata*, and Radix bupleurum, administered once in the morning and once in the evening. The therapeutic effects were evaluated after eight weeks of treatment. The results revealed a clinically effective rate of 94.29% in the treatment group, significantly surpassing that of the control group. Following treatment, the scores for TCM symptoms such as epigastric distension and pain, chest and hypochondriac distension and pain, emotional discomfort, epigastric noise, belching, acid reflux, dry mouth, bitter taste, and sticky stool were notably reduced in both groups. Furthermore, the scores and total scores of various traditional Chinese medicine symptoms in the treatment group were lower than those in the control group after treatment. According to these researchers, Almonds in Modified Sanren Decoction promote Qi movement and dampness elimination; Cardamom seed regulates Qi and harmonizes the stomach; Coix seed fosters water retention and strengthens the spleen. Modern pharmacological studies have also indicated that Sanren Decoction can reduce the degree of gastric mucosal inflammation in chronic gastritis by regulating the differential expression of gastric mucosal proteins and lowering the levels of gastrin and gastric actin, resulting in improved clinical symptoms and signs.

Liu Chenping and Li Yiping [7] conducted a study involving 35 patients diagnosed with chronic atrophic gastritis to assess the clinical effectiveness of Anwei Decoction in treating the spleen deficiency and blood stasis type of chronic atrophic gastritis, along with its impact on the hemorheological indicators of patients. The traditional Chinese medicine composition of Anwei Decoction includes *Codonopsis pilosula*, Atractylodes macrocephala, Poria, Scutellaria baicalensis, tangerine peel, Radix Glycyrrhizae, and others. After three months of treatment, the researchers observed the TCM syndrome scores and hemorheology indexes of both groups. The results revealed that following treatment, the overall clinical effective rate in the treatment group was 91.4%, surpassing that of the control group (80.6%). The TCM syndrome score in the treatment group was lower than that in the control group, and the treatment group exhibited better therapeutic effects in terms of enhancing whole blood reductive viscosity, plasma viscosity, erythrocyte sedimentation rate, and erythropoiesis equality. This suggests that Anwei Decoction could enhance blood flow status in patients, improve local blood supply, and facilitate the repair of gastric mucosa. The researchers posit that *Codonopsis pilosula* in Anwei Decoction strengthens the spleen and replenishes Qi. When combined with Atractylodes macrocephala, Poria cocos, and Radix Glycyrrhizae, it forms Sijunzi Decoction, amplifying its spleen-tonifying effects. A healthy spleen promotes adequate circulation of Qi and blood, ensuring unobstructed Qi mechanisms.

Years of clinical research and pharmacological investigations have revealed that Xiangsha Liujunzi Decoction, in the treatment of gastrointestinal diseases, can enhance gastrointestinal motility, alleviate spasticity, reduce gastrointestinal mucosal inflammation, and exert a positive influence on gastric mucosa, flora, and small intestinal motility [8]. In a study conducted by Liu Xia [9], 47 patients with chronic atrophic gastritis were enrolled to evaluate the clinical effectiveness of Xiangsha Liujunzi Decoction in treating chronic gastritis. The control group received conventional Western medicine treatment, while the treatment group was administered Xiangsha Liujunzi Decoction. This prescription includes Atractylodes macrocephala, Poria cocos, *Codonopsis pilosula*, Tangerine peel, Radix Glycyrrhizae Preparata, Amomum villosum, among other ingredients. After two months of treatment, the results revealed that the treatment group receiving Xiangsha Liujunzi Decoction had significantly lower scores for symptoms such as epigastric pain or flatulence, shortness of breath, lazy speech, and loose stool compared to the control group. Moreover, the treatment group exhibited lower scores for gastric mucosal atrophy and intestinal metaplasia compared to the control group. Researchers believe that Amomum villosum in Xiangsha Liujunzi Decoction plays a protective role in gastric mucosa by exerting anti-inflammatory effects and inhibiting platelet aggregation. *Pinellia ternata* can alleviate cough, phlegm, vomiting, inhibit inflammatory reactions, and impede the development of gastric cancer cells. Tangerine peel offers antioxidant, antibacterial, and immune-regulatory properties, while also reducing blood lipid levels and demonstrating anti-tumor effects. These findings demonstrate the favorable therapeutic effect of Xiangsha Liujunzi Decoction on chronic atrophic gastritis, effectively relieving clinical symptoms and signs while reducing inflammatory damage to the gastric mucosa.

Collectively, the aforementioned clinical trials underscore the substantial advantages of traditional Chinese medicine in the treatment of chronic gastritis. It offers high safety and minimal side effects, effectively improving the clinical symptoms, controlling and reversing gastric mucosal atrophy, reducing recurrence, and decreasing the transformation rate to gastric cancer. As such, it stands as a reliable, safe, and valuable complementary and alternative therapy.

3. Acupuncture and moxibustion, massage for chronic gastritis

3.1 Acupuncture

In clinical practice, chronic gastritis patients are predominantly treated with pharmaceuticals. However, these drugs often come with significant side effects and should not be used over extended periods. Acupuncture, as a treatment for chronic gastritis, offers notable improvements in patients' clinical symptoms and is gaining increasing attention in research.

Acupoints represent specialized locations along the meridians that carry the flow of qi and blood within the body's internal organs. They also serve as reaction points for diseases and focal points for acupuncture and other therapeutic interventions. Clinical experiments examining pain-sensitive points in patients with chronic non-atrophic gastritis (CNAG) have revealed [10] that these patients commonly exhibit sensitivity at various acupoints. The most frequently affected meridians are the ren pulse, gastric meridian, spleen meridian, kidney meridian, bladder meridian, with some instances occurring outside meridians and non-acupoint areas. Acupuncture at these sensitivity points significantly alleviates the level of pain sensitivity experienced by patients. This improvement in pain sensitivity helps alleviate clinical symptoms such as stomach pain, abdominal fullness, heartburn, acid reflux, belching, and more. Research has indicated that acupoint pain sensitivity is linked to the sensitization of spinal cord dorsal horn neurons by internal organs. This sensitization leads to a heightened response of neurons to signals originating from the body's surface. Each organ corresponds to a specific nerve segment, making pain-sensitive points commonly located within the nerve segment innervating the organ or adjacent nerve segment areas.

Acupuncture, a method involving the use of a red-hot needle, quickly punctures the selected point or area with the aid of the dual stimulation of acupuncture and heat. A clinical study conducted at the First Affiliated Hospital of Tianjin University of Chinese Medicine [11] employed fire acupuncture (0.4 × 35 mm) for rapid puncture in the treatment group. The results demonstrated that fire acupuncture significantly improved symptoms like stomach fullness, stomach pain, chest and hypochondrium pain, poor feeding, nausea, and vomiting in patients with chronic gastritis (CG). Moreover, patients' physiological and psychological well-being saw significant improvement following fire acupuncture treatment. It effectively alleviated anxiety and depression in CG patients and enhanced their overall quality of life.

Zhou Wei et al. [12] conducted a comparative study to assess the effectiveness of meridian diagnosis and acupuncture against conventional acupuncture in treating CAG. The observation group employed a comprehensive approach, utilizing meridian energy analyzers and hand inspection meridian methods to identify and select meridian points. They also selected the plus Luo-connecting point and Back-Shu point empirically and made adjustments to the points of eight extra meridians following acupuncture principles. In contrast, the control group primarily used acupoints including Zhongwan (RN12), Neiguan (PC6), Zusanli (ST36), and Gongsun (SP4) based on dialectical considerations. The results indicated that meridian diagnosis and acupuncture were superior to conventional acupuncture in treating CAG. This approach produced more significant effects on the pathology of gastric mucosa and maintained stable long-term efficacy.

Acupuncture, when applied in the treatment of CG, has demonstrated positive clinical outcomes by inhibiting inflammatory factors, protecting the gastric mucosa, and enhancing patients' quality of life. However, certain challenges exist, including the limited scale of research that may affect its credibility. Moreover, different pathological types and traditional Chinese medicine symptom types require distinct treatment approaches, and the criteria for assessing efficacy lack uniformity, diminishing the comparability of various studies. To address these issues, future studies should focus on increasing sample sizes in experimental and clinical research to enhance the credibility of their findings.

3.2 Moxibustion

Moxibustion, a traditional therapeutic technique in Chinese medicine, is renowned for its ability to stimulate acupoints along the body's meridians, warming them, dispelling cold, alleviating pain, and reducing swelling [13]. It has shown significant effectiveness in improving clinical symptoms of patients suffering from CG and positively impacting abnormal pathological manifestations of the gastric mucosa. Chinese medicine encompasses a variety of traditional moxibustion methods. This section focuses on the current research related to commonly used moxibustion techniques in the clinical treatment of CG.

Mild moxibustion falls within the category of suspended moxibustion, using moxa sticks. In this method, the ignited end of the moxa stick is held approximately an inch away from the skin at the moxibustion site, providing patients with a warm sensation without causing burning pain. Xie Hua et al. observed the clinical effectiveness of mild moxibustion in treating superficial gastritis with spleen and stomach deficiency-cold syndrome. They found that mild moxibustion can improve clinical symptoms in patients and regulate the levels of serum prostaglandin E2 (PGE2), somatostatin (SS), and epidermal growth factor (EGF). Moreover, it has shown long-term efficacy. The team also investigated the varying therapeutic effects of different moxibustion durations for this condition and discovered that mild moxibustion for 20 minutes significantly alleviates gastric pain, while mild moxibustion for 40 minutes has a more pronounced effect on relieving upper abdominal distension symptoms [14, 15].

Grain-sized moxibustion involves applying moxibustion by placing small pieces of moxa floss, approximately the size of a wheat grain, on the skin. The combustion temperature is carefully controlled to ensure optimal efficacy. This method promotes the flow of energy, activates the body's defense mechanisms, and enhances immune function. Cai Yumei and colleagues [16] observed that grain-sized moxibustion significantly improves symptom scores in patients with chronic superficial gastritis (CSG) and enhances their overall physiological and psychological quality of life scores (PCS and MCS). This technique effectively improves the clinical symptoms and quality of life of CSG patients, with better long-term efficacy compared to warm needle moxibustion. Liu Xiaofeng [17] and others used modified painless grain-sized septic moxibustion combined with traditional Chinese medicine to treat chronic non-atrophic gastritis (CNAG). This approach not only effectively improved the clinical symptoms of CNAG patients but also significantly enhanced their quality of life. The long-term efficacy of this combined treatment surpassed that of traditional Chinese medicine alone. Septic moxibustion, a distinctive therapy in traditional Chinese medicine, stimulates the body's immune response through the persistent local inflammatory reaction generated during the treatment process [18].

Ginger partition moxibustion is a moxibustion method that involves placing thin slices of ginger as a barrier on the moxibustion site. Ginger's spicy flavor and mild warming properties are harnessed to enhance the warmth generated during moxibustion. This technique stimulates meridian points in the human body, enhancing stomach motility, regulating gastric protease and gastric acid levels, and inhibiting gastric inflammatory reactions. It can also improve gastric mucosal atrophy and intestinal transformation [19]. Cao Wen [20] further improved the clinical effectiveness of treating CAG by adding ginger partition moxibustion to conventional Western medicine. This approach alleviated symptoms such as stomach distension and pain while protecting the gastric mucosa and reducing atrophy. He Jing [21] compared the clinical effectiveness of traditional moxibustion sticks and smokeless moxibustion sticks with ginger partition moxibustion in CAG treatment. Both methods significantly improved clinical symptoms and regulated serum indicators such as gastric secretin CAS. Traditional moxibustion sticks provided better efficacy due to their longer suitable temperature and stimulation time compared to smokeless moxibustion sticks with ginger partition moxibustion. Additionally, Yi Zhan et al. investigated the effects of different durations of ginger-separated moxibustion on the levels of superoxide dismutase (SOD) and malondialdehyde (MDA) in the serum of patients with chronic superficial gastritis and spleen and stomach deficiency-cold syndrome. The results demonstrated that ginger-separated moxibustion increased the activity of the antioxidant enzyme SOD while decreasing the levels of the free radical MDA in the serum. Furthermore, compared to ginger-separated moxibustion lasting for 20 minutes, ginger-separated moxibustion for 40 minutes had a significantly greater effect on increasing SOD levels. This suggests that the therapeutic effect of ginger-separated moxibustion in treating chronic gastritis may be associated with its positive regulation of the enzyme system involved in the production and clearance of oxygen free radicals [22].

Medicinal cakes used in partition moxibustion are typically composed of warm and pungent herbs such as Aconiti Radix and Cinnamomi Ramulus. When subjected to the heat produced during moxibustion, the active ingredients in these medicinal cakes are absorbed through the skin. This method avoids potential liver damage that can occur with oral medication metabolism. Gu Mu'en [23] conducted a comparison between the treatment of CAG patients using partition moxibustion with medicinal cakes and ginger partition moxibustion. The results indicated that both methods improved clinical symptoms in CAG patients and alleviated gastric mucosal atrophy and intestinal transformation. The use of medicinal cakes in partition moxibustion had advantages in improving symptoms like stomach pain and decreased appetite.

Moxa box moxibustion involves inserting moxa into a special moxa box placed in corresponding parts for moxibustion. The use of moxa boxes concentrates the heat generated by burning moxa sticks, maintaining a consistent moxibustion temperature and fully leveraging the warming and tonifying effects on the body's deficiencies and qi and blood. Wang Xiaowen [24] employed box moxibustion combined with herbal warm compress to treat chronic gastritis patients, resulting in significant alleviation of epigastric pain and improved clinical efficacy.

In conclusion, moxibustion therapy has demonstrated significant effectiveness and safety in treating chronic gastritis. In the future, further exploration of various moxibustion techniques for gastritis treatment, including acupuncture point selection, clinical procedures, and therapeutic effects, can be conducted to establish standards. This will hold greater significance for guiding scientific research and clinical practice.

3.3 Massage therapy for chronic gastritis

The vibration method is a commonly employed massage technique in clinical practice, known for its positive therapeutic effects on spleen and stomach diseases along with their accompanying symptoms and complications. In the vibration method, the entire palm, base of the palm, or fingertip of the finger serves as the focal point. It generates tremors through small and rapid alternating contractions and relaxations of the forearm flexor and extensor muscles, transmitting force to the deeper parts of the body [25].

Abdominal vibration massage is a commonly used massage technique in the clinical treatment of chronic gastritis [26]. This method focuses on the abdominal Shenque acupoint and involves stimulating various meridians, including the Ren meridian, kidney meridian, spleen, and stomach meridian. It induces stable and continuous tremors, triggering biochemical reactions and neurohumoral changes in the body. This approach helps regulate immune function, improve physiological functioning, and contribute to disease treatment. When combined with abdominal massage, it effectively regulates the middle energizer and the three energizer passageways, which is essential for balancing spleen and stomach qi function in the treatment of chronic gastritis. Effective treatment of chronic gastritis revolves around maintaining the balance of spleen and stomach qi. This balance is achieved through mechanical and warm stimulation that promotes the absorption of gastric mucosal inflammation, ulcer repair, and disease control. The abdominal vibration massage method focuses on the abdomen, using the Shenque acupoint at the palm's root as the center. It gently and continuously vibrates, stimulating the spleen and stomach meridians of the middle energizer and both sides. During the procedure, practitioners can also apply pressure to the Qihai (RN6), Tianshu (ST25), and Zhongwan (RN12). Chronic gastritis often has a connection to liver depression, and patients' clinical symptoms are frequently linked to emotional fluctuations. The abdominal vibration massage method targets the Shenque acupoint as the center and stimulates the Belt Vessel and Tianshu acupoints on both sides through gentle rhythmic vibrations. This helps unblock liver and gallbladder qi, regulate the central nervous system, promote qi circulation, alleviate depression, clear the intestines, and enhance gastrointestinal peristalsis. Additionally, abdominal rubbing and kneading techniques generate heat and drive subcutaneous tissue, benefiting individuals with severe Qi stagnation. Yi Liujuan [27] conducted research on the effect of the palm vibration method as the primary massage technique combined with stellate ganglion catgut embedding for improving clinical symptoms in patients with chronic gastritis. The results indicated that single catgut embedding treatment was slower in its effect. However, when combined with the palm vibration method, it significantly improved traditional Chinese medicine symptoms, clinical symptoms, and reduced oxidative stress reactions in patients with chronic gastritis. This combination therapy demonstrated enhanced efficacy in alleviating chronic gastritis symptoms.

The back massage method is often employed to treat chronic gastritis, especially in cases where patients exhibit spleen and stomach deficiency, an inability to transform their diet, or damage to the middle yang. Chronic gastritis of this nature may manifest as endogenous deficiency and cold, bloating, pain, a gradual loss of spleen and stomach transformation, a decline in spleen yang, and even involvement of kidney yang. In such cases, all organs lack nourishment. Abdominal vibration massage, when used in this context, targets the Shenque acupoint and stimulates the meridians, navel circumference, and vital gate. It strengthens the central area while nourishing the fire and soil, promoting warmth and nourishment in the body. Jiang Manjun [28] also suggested that massage therapy can be beneficial for individuals with chronic superficial gastritis of the spleen-stomach deficiency cold type. The treatment involves using the thumb or middle finger's abdominal force to massage specific parts or acupoints on the abdomen and back, focusing on the Governor Vessel and back shu acupoints. This approach follows the theory of acupoint matching between back-shu points and front-mu points and interacts with abdominal and Conception Vessel acupoints, which are related to corresponding organs. By infusing Yang Qi into each organ, it stimulates Yang Qi distribution throughout the body via the meridians. This ensures the normal operation and gasification function of organs like the spleen and stomach. Li Nanxi [29] and others have also demonstrated that massaging along the meridians on the abdomen and back can clear the meridians, regulate yin and yang, strengthen the spleen and stomach, and promote qi regulation. This approach has shown promise in treating chronic gastritis.

In summary, patients treated with the vibration massage as the primary method have experienced significant improvements in clinical symptoms such as loss of appetite, bloating, abdominal pain, belching, and pantothenic acid. In clinical practice, SOD and MDA are commonly used oxidative stress indicators [30]. The massage method, particularly the vibration method, changes the internal environment's state through stimulation. Techniques like pressing, pressing, and rubbing unblock the meridians, enhance gastrointestinal motility, and significantly reduce oxidative stress reactions. Overall, massage treatment for chronic gastritis has demonstrated favorable therapeutic effects and promising applications.

4. Diet therapy for chronic gastritis

Diet therapy plays a significant role in the management of chronic gastritis. TCM diet therapy utilizes the principles of TCM to strengthen the body's resistance and eliminate pathogenic factors. In Chinese culture, there has long been an understanding that "medicine and food are homologous," emphasizing the idea that food can have therapeutic effects similar to medicine.

Chronic gastritis is a type of epigastric pain in traditional Chinese medicine (TCM). As the saying goes, "Treating the stomach requires three parts treatment and seven parts nourishment." Treating chronic gastritis involves adopting sensible dietary habits. Several studies have indicated that by understanding the causes of chronic gastritis and combining medication with dietary control, patients can alleviate symptoms and manage the disease's progression [31–33]. In recent years, a growing body of clinical data has affirmed that nourishing the spleen and stomach through diet benefits gastrointestinal function and is a crucial approach for treating and caring for chronic gastritis.

Wang Shurong et al. [34] adhere to TCM dietotherapy principles in clinical practice, providing tailored treatments based on patients' unique conditions. They conducted a study involving 60 patients with CAG. The control group received a regular diet, while the treatment group received a regular diet combined with dietotherapy based on syndrome differentiation. In TCM, CAG is categorized into various syndromes, including Deficiency-cold syndrome of spleen and stomach, Stomach Yin Deficiency Syndrome, Syndrome of stagnation of heat in the liver and stomach, Syndrome of blood stasis blocking the stomach, and Syndrome of food stagnation. Food materials are classified according to meridians for balanced compatibility, with corresponding treatments such as dried ginger porridge with yam, Adenophora ginseng and lily porridge, *Ophiopogon japonicus* porridge, Hawthorn and Tremella Soup, and Divine Comedy and Grain Sprout Porridge. The results revealed that the treatment group achieved an overall response rate of 95.0%, significantly higher than the control group's 83.3%, demonstrating the effectiveness of dialectical dietary therapy in improving chronic atrophic gastritis.

Wang Zhenzhen et al. [35] assert that, prior to commencing dietary nursing interventions, it is crucial to comprehensively explain the significance of dietary adjustments to patients. The research encompassed 110 patients suffering from chronic gastritis. The control group received standard nursing care, while the observation group had tailored dietary nursing strategies devised based on their specific syndrome types. For individuals with a Deficiency of spleen and stomach, the recommendation included consuming more easily digestible foods such as porridge, which nourishes the spleen and boosts qi, while also warming the stomach and dispelling cold sensations. These foods encompass millet, carrots, yams, etc. Conversely, they were advised to steer clear of cold and refrigerated fruits, as well as raw or chilled beverages like watermelon and bitter gourd. Patients exhibiting disharmony between the liver and stomach were directed to prioritize liquid and pasta-based meals, emphasizing slow chewing and swallowing, in addition to adhering to regular meal schedules. During their nursing period, abstaining from smoking or alcohol was encouraged, along with the consumption of foods conducive to stomach comfort and qi regulation, such as lotus root, lentils, and hawthorn, while avoiding fatty and heavy fare such as greasy meats and seafood, etc. For those with damp-heat type spleen and stomach conditions, an intake rich in heat-clearing, diuretic, yin-nourishing, and fluid-promoting foods, like lotus seeds, red beans, cucumbers, etc., was suggested. On the flip side, spicy and fiery foods, such as pepper and ginger, were to be avoided. Patients exhibiting stomach yin deficiency were advised to include more qi-replenishing, yin-nourishing, and moisture-enhancing foods in their diets, like duck, milk, tremella, and lily, while steering clear of items known to generate heat and harm yin, such as mutton, dog meat, strong tea, coffee, and garlic, etc. Those with blood stasis in stomach collaterals were encouraged to consume foods promoting qi and blood circulation, including eggplant, kelp, and mushrooms, while avoiding astringent and cold items like dark plum, sweet potatoes, and persimmons, etc. Furthermore, it was recommended to prompt patients to diligently record their daily dietary choices, meal times, and meal frequency. Healthcare professionals should maintain continuous monitoring of the patients' adherence to their dietary plans and offer timely, tailored guidance. The results demonstrated that, in comparison to the control group, patients in the observation group experienced a shorter duration of upper abdominal pain, abdominal distension, and other adverse symptoms. They also reported greater satisfaction and exhibited improved nutritional status. This study underscores that judicious application of dietary therapy as an adjunctive treatment in patients with chronic atrophic gastritis serves not only as nutritional support but also as a therapeutic measure. Additionally, it can enhance patients' quality of life and satisfaction with nursing care. Dietary therapy effectively merges prevention and treatment, yielding satisfactory therapeutic outcomes and showcasing the distinctive facets of TCM dietary practices.

Liu Jun [36] emphasizes the limitations of single-drug therapy and underscores the importance of incorporating diet therapy into the treatment of chronic gastritis alongside peptic ulcers. This study involved 82 patients with both chronic gastritis and peptic ulcers. In this approach, physicians are advised not only to guide patients in taking omeprazole capsules regularly and in appropriate doses but also to offer dietary recommendations tailored to the patient's clinical symptoms and condition. A scientifically sound dietary plan should be devised to encourage the consumption of low-fat, high-protein, and easily digestible foods. It is recommended to include items such as cucumber, cabbage, apples, pears, and to consume warm water before meals, which can effectively safeguard the gastric mucosa.

Mao Yanping et al. [37, 38] have established a strong connection between dietary cellulose intake and dietary habits with CAG (chronic atrophic gastritis). A high dietary fiber diet has demonstrated the ability to delay or even reverse the progression of this disease. Zheng Jie, and others [39] contend that many high dietary fiber sources exhibit excellent anti-inflammatory and antioxidant properties, with common sources being legumes, seaweed, mushrooms, fruits, vegetables, and rhizomes. Notably, seaweed boasts the highest dietary fiber content, followed by grains, mushrooms, roots, fruits, and vegetables. Building upon this, Zhu Chunhua and Feng Yuke [40] conducted a group intervention and observation study involving 86 CAG patients to investigate the application of a high-fiber diet. The results demonstrated that after the intervention, both groups experienced improvements in mental health, physiological function, emotional well-being, and social function, with the observation group showing greater improvements. This highlights the significant impact of a high-fiber diet on CAG patients, enhancing their condition, nutritional status, and overall quality of life.

Gao Fan [41] conducted a review of clinical data from 80 children with chronic gastritis to assess the effectiveness of seamless nursing combined with diet intervention. Nutritionists crafted personalized dietary plans based on the child's age and condition. These plans included foods rich in fiber, protein, vitamins, and zinc, such as eggs, lotus root, carrots, and shrimp. Additionally, easily digestible and light foods like broccoli, noodles, and bananas were recommended, while hard, overheated, excessively cold, highly acidic, spicy, or greasy foods were discouraged. Guidance on developing healthy eating habits, including chewing slowly, consuming smaller, more frequent meals, and avoiding overeating, was provided. The results indicate that, alongside effective chronic gastritis treatment, it is essential to create a scientifically rational dietary plan tailored to the child's condition. This approach helps alleviate clinical symptoms and enhance compliance. Dietary intervention effectively assists children with chronic gastritis in forming healthy eating habits, ensuring adequate nutrition during treatment, promoting physical recovery, and bolstering overall health [42, 43].

Lu Meirong and Zheng Shufeng [44, 45] both stress the significance of dietary intervention and dietary health education in caring for patients with chronic gastritis. Zheng conducted a study with 56 chronic gastritis patients, dividing them into a control group and an observation group. The control group received standard care, while the observation group underwent specific dietary interventions, including the following steps: Firstly, doctors should guide patients in adapting their diet plans, emphasizing eating smaller, more frequent meals, and increasing the frequency of chewing during meals to enhance digestion. Secondly, it is essential to establish a rational dietary structure, encouraging patients to consume more vegetables and foods rich in vitamins that are easily digestible and highly nutritious. Cooking methods should primarily involve steaming, boiling, stewing, and braising, while methods such as frying and roasting should be avoided. Legumes and peanuts should be cooked before consumption. Lastly, attention should be devoted to dietary hygiene, avoiding overeating and refraining from consuming spicy, irritating, and cold foods to prevent aggravation of the condition due to irritation of the gastric mucosa. For patients experiencing symptoms like nausea, vomiting, and acute massive bleeding, it is advisable to abstain from eating. For patients with peptic ulcers, a diet consisting of mild and liquid foods is recommended after 12–24 hours of bleeding cessation. In the case of cirrhosis patients, they should opt for liquid foods rich in vitamins and high in calories after 2–3 days of bleeding cessation, while strictly limiting sodium, salt, and protein intake. These research findings indicate that dietary care serves a dual purpose: on one hand, it helps mitigate the gastrointestinal burden resulting from poor dietary habits, which can stimulate gastric mucosal function and exacerbate the condition; on the other hand, it provides essential nutrients for recovery, facilitating disease improvement. Effective management of chronic gastritis cannot be divorced from sound dietary practices. The integration of dietary intervention with health education not only prevents and treats chronic gastritis but also enhances patients' psychological well-being, sleep quality, quality of life, and daily functioning, while also reducing the risk of disease recurrence. It stands as a vital measure in the treatment and care of chronic gastritis.

The clinical trial results mentioned above demonstrate the effectiveness of dietary therapy in enhancing the well-being of chronic gastritis patients. It effectively alleviates adverse symptoms like nausea and vomiting, boosts patients' psychological health, elevates nutritional levels, mitigates complications arising from nutritional deficiencies during treatment, enhances patients' quality of life, and improves their overall physical condition. This underscores that dietary therapy is a dependable, efficient, and secure complementary treatment option deserving of widespread clinical adoption and utilization.

5. Chronic gastritis exercise alternative therapy

Chronic gastritis is primarily characterized by symptoms like epigastric pain, abdominal bloating, and indigestion. Engaging in appropriate and moderate exercise can have several positive effects on gastrointestinal health. It can enhance gastrointestinal peristalsis, improve blood circulation to the gastric mucosa, facilitate the healing of gastric mucosal inflammation, and consequently enhance digestive function and stimulate appetite. Additionally, regular physical activity can alleviate symptoms of anxiety, depression, and loneliness often experienced by chronic gastritis patients. Moreover, it contributes to the maintenance of a balanced yin and yang within the body. In traditional Chinese medicine, the practice of gongfu exercises is known to boost yang qi, regulate the flow of qi and blood, strengthen the body, and enhance the body's ability to prevent diseases [46].

A survey conducted by Deng Tietao, a master of Traditional Chinese medicine, examined 147 individuals. It found that 64 individuals "felt that their spleen and stomach functions were normal," of whom 60.94% (39/64) engaged in regular physical activity. In contrast, of the remaining 83 individuals who "felt that their spleen and stomach functions were not normal," 32.53% (27/83) engaged in regular physical activity. This survey explored public attitudes toward Chinese medicine exercise techniques, exercise habits, and gastrointestinal health. The findings suggest that individuals with normal spleen and stomach functions are more likely to be frequent physical exercisers, hinting at the potential benefits of exercise for spleen and stomach health. Research has shown that exercise has a bidirectional stimulating effect on gastrointestinal muscles, promoting gastrointestinal muscle peristalsis, enhancing the secretion of digestive juices, regulating cerebral intestinal peptides, and improving the body's microenvironment [47].

In a study by Wang Jing, 124 cases of bile reflux gastritis were randomly divided into a treatment group and a control group. The results revealed that combining exercise therapy with Western medicine for the treatment of bile reflux gastritis can improve clinical outcomes, offering valuable insights for clinical practice [48]. Traditional Chinese Medicine Guidance, a branch of exercise therapy, incorporates traditional techniques like the Eight-Section Brocade, Tai Chi, Five-Animal Exercise, and more. It emphasizes the integration of physical movement, breathing, and psychological regulation, focusing on regulating the body, breathing, and heart as fundamental elements. This approach has demonstrated clinical efficacy and research significance in preventing and treating diseases of the digestive system, cardiovascular system, and tumors [49]. Utilizing Traditional Chinese Medicine Guidance, such as the Eight-Section Brocade and Five-Animal Exercise, often yields positive therapeutic outcomes in the treatment of chronic gastritis.

Huang Lingshan conducted research on the treatment of chronic gastritis patients using Eight-Section Brocade Exercises. The treatment group exhibited significantly quicker pain reduction compared to the control group. Eight-Section Brocade Exercises, characterized as mild and safe aerobic exercise, play a role in harmonizing internal organs and achieving the goal of "stabilizing the five organs and stabilizing the blood vessels." This exercise, with its "rigid and flexible" movements, can effectively clear qi and blood meridians, regulate internal organ function, enhance physical fitness, improve the quality of life for patients with chronic gastritis and liver-stomach disharmony, and enhance the effectiveness of treatment [50]. Li Zhou and colleagues investigated the impact of Eight-Section Brocade on the care outcomes of patients with chronic gastritis accompanied by anxiety and depression. In the study, the control group received routine treatment and care, while the observation group incorporated the Eight-Section Brocade into their care regimen alongside routine treatment. The results revealed that the observation group experienced better therapeutic outcomes compared to the control group. The application of Eight-Section Brocade in the care of patients with chronic gastritis and comorbid anxiety and depression positively influenced their clinical symptoms and psychological well-being, thereby facilitating their recovery [51].

Zhang Ping researched the effects of Bear Exercise within the Five-Animal Exercise regimen on patients with chronic atrophic gastritis. The findings demonstrated that the addition of Bear Exercise to conventional treatment was more effective in alleviating gastrointestinal discomfort symptoms, with improvements becoming more pronounced over time [52].

Chronic gastritis, characterized by its enduring and recurrent nature due to multiple factors, benefits from exercise in improving and regulating organ function to establish a relative balance between yin and yang within the body. Experimental studies have revealed that exercise induces the cerebral cortex to enter an inhibitory state, facilitating the restoration of normal regulatory function in the central nervous system. This adjustment influences the activity of the autonomic nervous system, enhancing gastric peristalsis and diaphragmatic movement, which, in turn, promotes gastric juice secretion and an increase in salivary amylase content, thus boosting appetite and facilitating weight gain [53].

Consequently, regular exercise holds considerable benefits for patients with chronic gastritis, aiding in their recovery and overall well-being. Exercise serves as a pivotal component in the prevention and treatment of chronic gastritis and can serve as a valuable reference for clinical practice.

6. Psychological intervention therapy for chronic gastritis

Chronic gastritis, a prevalent gastrointestinal ailment, is chiefly characterized by upper abdominal pain, feelings of fullness and burning sensations, which tend to worsen after meals, significantly impacting the daily lives and work routines of affected individuals. The protracted treatment course and unpredictable nature of the condition can lead to persistent abdominal pain during the therapeutic process, subsequently giving rise to negative emotions such as anxiety, depression, pessimism, or tension among patients. Prolonged negative emotions can gradually precipitate psychological disorders, manifesting not only as gastrointestinal lesions stemming from gastritis but also encompassing symptoms like depression, irritability, and insomnia, further exacerbating the condition and impeding treatment effectiveness. In light of these challenges, it is recommended to complement the standard treatment of chronic gastritis with essential psychological interventions aimed at mitigating adverse psychological states and enhancing patient treatment compliance.

In a recent clinical study involving 77 patients grappling with chronic gastritis [54], a noteworthy distinction became evident between two distinct groups. When compared to the control cohort, which solely received fundamental care measures, the experimental group underwent a comprehensive regimen encompassing individualized dietary guidance and behavioral psychological interventions. The results were remarkable: the experimental group exhibited significantly reduced levels of anxiety, depression, and pain. Simultaneously, they experienced substantial enhancements in social interactions, sleep quality, and emotional well-being. These findings underscore the significant potential of individualized dietary care and behavioral psychological interventions in augmenting the efficacy of chronic gastritis treatment, ultimately elevating the overall quality of life for patients.

In another clinical study conducted at the Zhengzhou Hospital of Traditional Chinese Medicine [55], 61 patients diagnosed with chronic gastritis were randomly divided into two groups. The control group (n = 30) received standard care, while the study group (n = 31) received standard care coupled with comprehensive psychological support. This support encompassed mental health assessments, empathetic listening, health education, mindfulness-based silence therapy, cognitive and emotional therapy, as well as verbal and non-verbal communication. Following the intervention, it became evident that the study group, in comparison to the control group, exhibited superior improvements in SAS and SDS scores. Additionally, the study group demonstrated a notably higher treatment compliance rate (96.77%) when contrasted with the control group (73.33%). This study underscores the potential advantages of integrating comprehensive psychological care with standard treatment to assist patients in managing their emotional well-being, rectifying misconceptions, and enhancing treatment compliance.

The clinical study results mentioned above consistently highlight the significant advantages of incorporating psychological interventions, which are inherently safe. These interventions efficiently alleviate negative emotions in chronic gastritis patients, improve treatment adherence, and notably alleviate the clinical symptoms associated with this condition. As such, they represent a dependable, safe, and complementary therapeutic approach that merits broader promotion and adoption.

Author details

Liu Mi[1*], Liu Weiai[2], She Chang[3], Zhou Jingying[1], Xu Xuan[1] and He Haolong[1]

1 College of Acupuncture, Tuina and Rehabilitation, Hunan University of Chinese Medicine, Changsha, China

2 The Second Affiliated Hospital of Hunan University of Chinese Medicine, Changsha, China

3 Changsha Hospital of Traditional Chinese Medicine, Changsha, China

*Address all correspondence to: 7417091@qq.com

References

[1] Tian G, Wu C, Li J, et al. Network pharmacology based investigation into the effect and mechanism of modified Sijunzi decoction against the subtypes of chronic atrophic gastritis. Pharmacological Research. 2019;**144**:158-166

[2] Zhao YS. Clinical analysis of modified Banxia Xiexin decoction in the treatment of chronic atrophic gastritiswith cold-heat complicated syndrome. Chinese Journal of Modern Drug Application. 2023;**17**(13):148-150

[3] Ma CL, Xiao JC, Wang Y, et al. Clinical study of Moluodan combined with hydrotalcite in treatment of chronic atrophic gastritis. Drugs Clin. 2023;**38**(07):1702-1706

[4] Yu B, Huang LQ, Gao Y, et al. Dhase IV clinical trial of ligi Nuanwei granules in the treatment of chronic superficial gastritis. The Chinese Journal of Clinical Pharmacology. 2020;**36**(22):3608-3611

[5] Hu CP, Cai YS, Yang W, et al. Curative effect analysis of Pingwei decoction in the treatment of 60 cases of chronic gastritis atrophy and intestinal metaplasia. Journal of Sichuan Traditional Chinese Medicine. 2021;**39**(05):102-104

[6] Guo XY, Liu CX, Zhao D, et al. Clinical efficacy of modified Sanren decoction for chronic non-atrophic gastritis of spleendeficiency damp-heat and liver stagnation. Hebei Journal of Traditional Chinese Medicine. 2023;**45**(07):1097-1101

[7] Liu CP, Li YP. Efficacy of modified Anwei decoction in treating chronic atrophic gastritis patients with syndromeof spleen deficiency and blood stasis and its influence on hemorheology. Acta Universitatis Traditionis Medicalis Sinensis Pharmacologiaeque Shanghai. 2019;**33**(01):28-31

[8] Wang J, Song N, Chen S, et al. Effect and mechanism of Xiangsha Liujunzi decoction on hepatic triglyceride synthesis in spleen deficiency hyperlipidemia rats based on the regulation of TMAO/perk/FoxO1 pathway by intestinal flora. Lishizhen Medicine And Materia Medica Research. 2022;**33**(02):286-291

[9] Liu X. Clinical observation of Xiangsha Liujunzi decoction in the treatment of chronic atrophic gastritis with spleen and stomach weakness syndrome. Journal of Traditional Chinese Medicine. 2023;**39**(07):1279-1282

[10] Zhang RY. Clinical Study on Acupuncture Treatment of Chronic Non-atrophic Gastritis Based on Acupoint Sensitization Theory. Kunming, Yunnan, China: Department of Acupuncture and Spleen and Gastroenterology, Yunnan Hospital of Traditional Chinese Medicine; 2021

[11] Liu ZG. Clinical Evaluation Study on the Improvement of Clinical Symptoms and Psychological Status of Chronic Gastritis Patients by Fire Acupuncture. Tianjin, China: Department of Acupuncture Six Wards and Outpatient Clinic, The First Affiliated Hospital of Tianjin University of Chinese Medicine; 2023

[12] Zhou W, Li YX, Zhang YX, et al. Observations on the efficacy of acupuncture in the treatment of chronic atrophic gastritis by meridian diagnosis and acupoint taking method. Chinese Acupuncture

and Moxibustion. 2020;**40**(09):928-932. DOI: 10.13703/j.0255-2930.20190717-k0005

[13] Xia ZL. Discussion on the drug basis of moxibustion efficacy in Chinese medicine and its mechanism of action. Journal of Chinese Medicine. 2015;**30**(02):297-299

[14] Xie H, Chang XR Yan J, et al. Clinical observation on superficial gastritis of deficient cold of spleen and stomach type treated by mild moxibustion. Chinese Journal of Traditional Chinese Medicine. 2011;**26**(12):2856-2858

[15] Xie H, Liu M, Chang XR, et al. Clinical observation on therapeutic effects of mild moxibustion in superficial gastritis patients with spleen-stomach deficiency-cold pattern. Acupuncture Research. 2012;**37**(04):318-323. DOI: 10.13702/j.1000-0607.2012.04.013

[16] Cai YM, Lu XJ, Zheng JF, et al. Clinical observation of wheat grain moxibustion in the treatment of spleen and stomach cold type chronic superficial gastritis. Chinese Acupuncture and Moxibustion. 2021;**41**(05):511-514

[17] Liu XF, Su XZ, Zhao DX, et al. The efficacy of modified painless wheat-grain septic moxibustion combined with traditional Chinese medicine in the treatment of chronic non-atrophic gastritis with spleen and stomach deficiency and cold. Shanghai Journal of Acupuncture and Moxibustion: 1-6

[18] Wei ZX, Zhang QL, Han L, et al. Clinical study on the treatment of cough variant asthma with modified painless wheat grain septic moxibustion. Shanghai Journal of Acupuncture and Moxibustion. 2021;**40**(06):658-663

[19] Jiang R, Yuan XK. Observation on the efficacy of internal administration of traditional Chinese medicine combined with ginger moxibustion for the treatment of Hp-positive chronic atrophic gastritis with intestinalization. China Clinical New Medicine. 2020;**13**(01):70-74

[20] Cao W, Zhang JJ, Lin CH, et al. Clinical study on the treatment of chronic atrophic gastritis by ginger moxibustion. Shanghai Journal of Acupuncture and Moxibustion. 2021;**40**(08):950-953

[21] He J, Li J, Gu ME, et al. Study on the therapeutic effect of ginger moxibustion with different moxibustion materials in the treatment of chronic atrophic gastritis. Shaanxi Traditional Chinese Medicine. 2022;**43**(06):797-800

[22] Yi Z, Liu M, Chang XR, et al. Influence of serum SOD and MDA by moxibustion on ginger therapy for chronic superficial gastritis spleen-stomach vacuity cold patients with different time. Chinese Journal of Experimental Prescriptions. 2012;**18**(23):301-304. DOI: 10.13422/j.cnki.syfjx. 2012.23.014

[23] Gu ME, Huang Y, Liu YN, et al. Clinical observation of moxibustion in the treatment of chronic atrophic gastritis and its effect on DNA methylation in peripheral blood. World TCM. 2022;**17**(03):295-303

[24] Wang XW, Kang LY, Zhang XF, et al. Study on the effect of moxibustion combined with traditional Chinese medicine and warm external application on chronic gastritis patients with cold spleen and stomach. Hebei Journal of Traditional Chinese Medicine. 2023;**38**(02):34-38

[25] Liang S, Gao JJ, Wang Z, et al. Research progress of vibration method. Journal of Chinese Medicine. 2020;**35**(02):291-294

[26] Hu KX, Zhou KL, Xue XN, et al. Discussion on the treatment of chronic gastritis by vibratory abdomen massage. Beijing Traditional Chinese Medicine. 2023;**42**(05):556-558

[27] Yi LJ. The effect of tuina combined with stellate ganglion threading on the improvement of clinical symptoms in patients with chronic gastritis. Journal of External Treatment of Traditional Chinese Medicine. 2021;**30**(03):50-52

[28] Wang J, Wang DQ. Meridian point abdominal and dorsal acupressure in the treatment of 35 cases of chronic superficial gastritis. Henan Traditional Chinese Medicine. 2015;**35**(10):2517-2518

[29] Li NX, Huang JJ, Huang ZX, et al. Progress of clinical research on abdominal and dorsal acupressure in the treatment of spleen and stomach diseases. Chinese Ethnic and Folk Medicine. 2021;**30**(01):82-86

[30] Lian David FLJ, Xu YF, et al. Establishment and evaluation of chronic gastritis model in helicobacter pylori-infected mice. Chinese journal of. Comparative Medicine. 2017;**27**(07):6-12

[31] Wang XN, Zhang YF, Xu CP. Progress in diagnosis and treatment of chronic atrophic gastritis. Central South Medical Science. 2020;**48**(03):323-326

[32] Sun A, Yu-Fong Chang J, Chiang CP. Smart link of chronic atrophic gastritis with atrophic glossitis, gastric parietal cell antibody positivity, vitamin B12 deficiency, and hyperhomocysteinemia. Journal of the Formosan Medical Association. 2020;**119**(5):1006-1007

[33] Jie C, Xing YQ. Observation on the effect of bismuth-containing quadruple therapy on chronic gastritis with positive Helicobacter pylori. Military Doctor. 2019;**62**(07):635-637

[34] Wang SR, Liu SZ. Clinical observation on 60 cases of chronic atrophic gastritis treated with Huoxue Qingwei decoction combined with syndrome differentiation dietotherapy. Hebei Traditional Chinese Medicine. 2015;**37**(09):1333-1335

[35] Zhang T, Wang ZZ. Application of traditional Chinese medicine diet nursing combined with auricular point burying beans in patients with chronic gastritis. Journal of Qilu Nursing. 2022;**28**(11):59-62

[36] Jun L. Efficacy of diet therapy combined with omeprazole in the treatment of chronic gastritis complicated with peptic ulcer. Guide to Chinese Medicine. 2021;**19**(09):102-103

[37] Mao YP. Application of personalized dietary intervention in elderly patients with chronic gastric ulcer. E-Journal of Practical Clinical Nursing. 2020;**5**(10):87

[38] Shen CF, Jiang Y. Dietary fiber meal replacement combined with low glycemic index medical food dietary management in patients with type 2 diabetes. Nursing Practice and Research. 2019;**16**(23):63-65

[39] Zheng J. Analysis of the intervention effect of dietary nursing on patients with gastritis and gastric ulcer. Gansu Science and Technology. 2020;**36**(02):126-128

[40] Zhu CH, Feng YK. Effect of high dietary fiber diet in patients with chronic atrophic gastritis. Clinical Medicine Research and Practice. 2022;**7**(27):57-59

[41] Gao F. Application of seamless care combined with dietary intervention in pediatric chronic gastritis. Practical Integrated Chinese and Western Medicine. 2022;**22**(17):118-120+124

[42] Zhao X, Wu M, Zhang D, et al. The relationship of interpersonal sensitivity

and depression among patients with chronic atrophic gastritis: The mediating role of coping styles. Journal of Clinical Nursing. 2018;**27**(5-6):e984-e991

[43] Xiao H, Zhao Z, Zhang C, et al. Influence of standardized nursing intervention combined with mindfulness stress reduction training on the curative effect, negative emotion, and quality of life in patients with chronic gastritis and gastric ulcer. Evidence-based Complementary and Alternative Medicine. 2021;**2021**:2131405

[44] Lu MR. The application value of dietary intervention combined with health education in the care of patients with chronic gastritis. Famous Doctors. 2022;**18**:129-131

[45] Zheng SF. Clinical study on chronic gastritis combined with TCM nursing. New Traditional Chinese Medicine. 2020;**52**(24):164-167

[46] Sha ZH, Wang JH, Wang Q, et al. Intervention strategy of home Chinese medicine diet exercise emotion behavior for chronic gastritis patients during the new crown epidemic. Modern Chinese Medicine. 2022;**42**(06):67-72

[47] Chang SQ, Liu WL, Hou ZK, et al. Exploration and analysis of the comprehensive sculling method of national medical master Deng Tietao for the prevention and treatment of gastrointestinal diseases. China Traditional Chinese Medicine Modern Distance Education. 2021;**19**(21):68-70

[48] Wang J. Exercise therapy combined with Western medicine for the treatment of bile reflux gastritis in 62 cases. Chinese Medicine Research. 2017;**30**(07):36-38

[49] Han XP, Tian SW, Dai JG, et al. Exploration of traditional Chinese medicine guided therapy for tumor related depression [J/OL]. Liaoning Journal of Traditional Chinese Medicine:1-10. Available from: http://h-p.kns.cnki.net.hnucm.opac.vip/kcms/detail/21.1128.R.20230210.1806.032.html [Accessed: September 5, 2023]

[50] Huang LS, Lin LY, Yu J. Application of eight-duan jin in 40 cases of liver-stomach disharmony type chronic gastritis. Fujian Traditional Chinese Medicine. 2017;**48**(06):71-72

[51] Li Z, Gao HM, Chen YF, Hong Y, Chen XY. The role of Ba Duan Jin in the care of patients with chronic gastritis accompanied by anxiety and depression. Chinese and Foreign Medical Research. 2020;**18**(07):118-120

[52] Zhang P, Xu CQ, Tao T, et al. Research on the application of bear play in patients with spleen and stomach qi deficiency type chronic atrophic gastritis. Chinese Nursing Journal. 2017;**52**(08):967-971

[53] Wenxu H. Qigong therapy for gastric diseases. Massage and Guidance. 1988;**05**:25-26 32

[54] Zhou X, Nie Y. Application value of individualized dietary care and behavioral psychological intervention in the treatment of chronic gastritis. World Digest of Recent Medical Information. 2019;**19**(45):266-267

[55] Liu Y. Application of psychological nursing in the treatment of chronic gastritis. Capital Food and Medicine. 2019;**26**(04):92